MANUAL
of
STUTTERING
INTERVENTION

Clinical Competence Series

Series Editor
Robert T. Wertz, Ph.D.
Lee Ann C. Golper, Ph.D.

The Effects of Drugs on Communication Disorders, 2nd Edition
Deanie Vogel, Ph.D., John E. Carter, M.D., and Phyllis B. Carter, Pharm.D.

Manual of Voice Treatment: Pediatrics to Geriatrics, 2nd Edition
Moya L. Andrews, Ed.D., CCC-SLP

Clinical Manual of Laryngectomy and
Head/Neck Cancer Rehabilitation, 2nd Edition
Janina K. Casper, Ph.D., and Raymond H. Colton, Ph.D.

Assessment and Intervention Resource for Hispanic Children
Hortencia Kayser, Ph.D.

Approaches to the Treatment of Aphasia
Nancy Helm-Estabrooks, Sc.D., and Audrey L. Holland, Ph.D.

Sourcebook for Medical Speech Pathology, 2nd edition
Lee Ann C. Golper, Ph.D., CCC-SLP

Developmental Reading Disabilities
Candance Goldsworthy, Ph.D.

Manual of Articulation and Phonological Disorders
Ken Bleile, Ph.D.

Right Hemisphere Communication Disorders:
Therapy and Management
Connie Tompkins, Ph.D., CCC-SLP

Videoendoscopy: From Velopharynx to Larynx
Michael P. Karnell, Ph.D.

Prosody Management of Communication Disorders
Patricia M. Hargrove, Ph.D., and Nancy S. McGarr, Ph.D.

Manual of Stuttering Intervention
Patricia M. Zebrowski, Ph.D., and Ellen M. Kelly, Ph.D.

MANUAL
of
STUTTERING
INTERVENTION

Patricia M. Zebrowski

Ellen M. Kelly

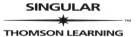

SINGULAR

THOMSON LEARNING

Australia Canada Mexico Singapore Spain United Kingdom United States

SINGULAR

---✦--- ™

THOMSON LEARNING

Manual of Stuttering Intervention
Patricia M. Zebrowski, Ph.D., and Ellen M. Kelly, Ph.D.

Singular Staff:

Healthcare Publishing
Director: William Brottmiller

Acquisitions Editor:
Candice Janco

Editorial Assistant:
Maria D'Angelico

Executive Marketing
Manager: Dawn Gerrain

Marketing Coordinator:
Kimberly Lourinia

Project Editor:
Mary Ellen Cox

Production Coordinator:
Anne Sherman

Art/Design Coordinator:
Jay Purcell

Library of Congress Cata-
loging-in-Publication Data

Zebrowski, Patricia M.
  Manual of stuttering
intervention / Patricia M.
Zebrowski, Ellen M. Kelly.
      p. cm.
  Includes bibliographical
references and index.
  ISBN 0-7693-0039-1
(alk. paper)
  1. Stuttering—Hand-
books, manuals, etc. I. Kelly,
Ellen M. II. Title.
  RC424 .Z43 2002
  616.85'54—dc21
                  2001042440

NOTICE TO THE READER

CONTENTS

FOREWORD

Com · pe · tence (kom' pə təns) n. The state or quality of being properly or well qualified; capable.

Clinicians crave competence. They pursue it through education and experience, through imitation and innovation. Regardless of the path taken to achieve clinical competence, there is nothing more useful than being guided by competent colleagues. This book, *Manual of Stuttering Intervention,* by Patricia Zebrowski and Ellen Kelly, demonstrates how combining the best empirical evidence with good old-fashioned clinical experience achieves the best practice. These two competent clinicians bring order and insight to appraising and mending disrupted fluency in children and adults. Both have a history of employing good science to advance our understanding of stuttering, and both are excellent examples of there being no substitute for hours of experience in the clinical trench. Drs. Zebrowski and Kelly emphasize the importance of the clients' perceptions about the way they talk and why consideration of these perceptions is essential in changing the way each client talks. The text abounds with case examples that demonstrate principles and application of techniques. Indeed, we are fortunate to have colleagues like Tricia Zebrowski and Ellen Kelly who have "been there, done that, and do it very well." Your attention to what they provide indicates your competence and your effort to improve it, because competent clinicians seek competence as much for what it demands, as for what it promises.

Robert T. Wertz, Ph.D.
Lee Ann C. Golper, Ph.D.
Series Editors

PREFACE

Developmental stuttering is a disorder of childhood that, for some, persists into adulthood. As the problem of stuttering develops over time, the speech behaviors that characterize it become layered with the individual's unique mix of learned and emotional responses, and those of family members. As such, the problem of stuttering has many dimensions that require the clinician's attention.

We wrote this book for students, for practicing clinicians who have limited experience working with adults and children who stutter, and for those experienced clinicians who are interested in brushing up on contemporary diagnostic and therapy strategies. We used the manual format so that the book will serve as an easy-to-access guide for the diagnosis and treatment of stuttering across the lifespan. In keeping with this manual (as opposed to textbook) format, our goal was to present a view of stuttering as the multilayered phenomenon that it is and to help clinicians to (1) identify and evaluate the contribution of each layer, and (2) solve the problem of how to address each in therapy. We tried to accomplish this through a combination of conceptual discussions about the intervention process and focused how-to descriptions of specific diagnostic and therapeutic techniques.

The manual is organized into six chapters. Chapter 1 addresses the issue of how to define stuttering and the very important differences between the ways in which clinicians define the term. Chapter 2 contains basic information for the assessment of stuttering, including our thoughts on how to interpret each piece of diagnostic information obtained. Chapter 3 presents an overview of the major approaches to the treatment of stuttering that are available today. In this chapter, we also provide some thoughts on the importance of the clinician's perspective; that is, what the clinician believes are the causes or contributing factors in the client's stuttering will determine the approaches used in therapy. Finally, we discuss some things to consider when setting the therapy agenda.

Chapters 4, 5, and 6 deal with the treatment of stuttering in preschool children, school-age children, and adults, respectively. These chapters provide the primary components to address specific treatments for each age group, and they offered the biggest challenge when we considered how to write them. Clearly, therapy for each age group could be the subject of an entire book or manual in itself. All challenges aside, however, the job of paring down information forces one to make (sometimes) hard decisions in choosing the fundamental concepts that cut across the entire spectrum of people who stutter, as well as the most salient issues relating to specific populations within the larger group. We both benefited from this "house cleaning," and we hope that you do as well!

ACKNOWLEDGMENTS

We would like to acknowledge our mentor, Edward G. Conture. He provided us with a model of professional excellence that has served as a strong foundation to our development as teachers, researchers, and clinicians. His dedication to mentoring doctoral students is unparalleled, and we thank him. We would also like to thank all of the clients with whom we have had the pleasure to work over the years. They have been, and continue to be, our best teachers. Finally, we would like to extend a special thanks to Sharon Thomason for her careful and timely assistance during the development of this manual.

DEDICATION

For all our past, present, and future students,
and for the many dedicated clinicians
who work with people who stutter.

You make a difference.

MANUAL
of
STUTTERING
INTERVENTION

CHAPTER

1

Definition of Stuttering

I. HOW DO WE DEFINE STUTTERING?

One of the first steps in developing a diagnostic and treatment plan for any communication disorder is to define the problem. This process provides the focus for clinical work, because it delineates the specific behaviors we want the client to acquire, eliminate, or change. Unfortunately, defining the problem is the clinician's most difficult task. Without a definition, speech-language pathologists may begin therapy not knowing where they are going or why.

A. Stuttering Can Be Defined as Both a Disorder and a Behavior

There can be different definitions for a speech or language problem, and it is sometimes difficult to know which definition will be the most beneficial for clinicians. This is certainly the case for stuttering—a problem that has a long history of debate over what is the *best* definition. For example, stuttering can be (and has been) defined broadly as a disorder of communication and, more specifically, as a behavior with observable and unobservable features.

1. **A Disorder.** Definitions of stuttering as a disorder deal with the etiology, or causes of stuttering, which are both proximal and distal. **Distal causes** result in the emergence or onset of stuttering in young children. **Proximal causes** trigger a moment or instance of stuttering by the person who stutters. According to Bloodstein (1995), distal causes of stuttering are explained by theories that were developed to describe the conditions under which stuttering first emerges in young children.

   Over the years, a number of such theories have been proposed, and naturally, they have influenced the clinical, decision-making process. For example, in his **diagnosogenic theory,** Johnson and others (1959) argued that stuttering in young children results from the child's attempts to avoid producing normal speech disfluencies which are evaluated by the child's parents to be stuttering. In this view, it is the parents' perception—not the child's speech—that is the primary contributing factor to the emergence of stuttering. Therefore, the parental thoughts, attitudes, and behaviors are the focal points in the evaluation and treatment of early stuttering. Later, Bloodstein (1975) proposed that stuttering in children develops as a reaction to the child's experience of chronic communicative failure. This suggests that a parent's negative evaluation of the child's speech, or the labeling of normal disfluency as stuttering, is only one example of such failure. Other potential causes may include the child's poor articulation, poor oral language skills, cognitive deficits, and verbal environment. In this **communicative failure–anticipatory struggle** hypothesis, a child who experiences chronic failure when attempting to communicate, for whatever reason, will anticipate difficulty in speaking situations. This anticipation, or sense of expectancy, will cause the child to use increased amounts of muscular tension while speaking, which ultimately leads to disfluency and stuttering. This theory broadened the number of factors considered important for the diagnosis and treatment of stuttering, and suggested that clinicians consider both the parents *and* the child as potential contributors to the onset and development of stuttering.

Theorists who attempt to explain the proximal causes of stuttering have argued that the moment, or instance, of stuttering is triggered by such factors as temporal discoordination of phonation with respiration and articulation (Perkins, Rudas, Johnson, & Bell, 1976; Kent, 1984); aberrant inputs to the muscles of speech production (Zimmermann, 1980); anticipatory avoidance (Johnson et al., 1967); and approach avoidance conflict (Sheehan, 1958). These theories, especially those that consider stuttered speech to be the end result of some breakdown or disruption in the temporal coordination of speech, have provided the framework for intervention approaches for the problem of stuttering. For example, "stutter more fluently" approaches in stuttering treatment emphasize the elimination of speech avoidance behaviors and fear reactions, while "speak more fluently" approaches focus on a relearning of the temporal patterns of nonstuttered speech. Integrated approaches utilize strategies from both schools of thought to speak and stutter more fluently, and add training in behavioral or physical awareness of the speech process.

Smith and Kelly (1997) have proposed a **multifactorial** view of stuttering in which they describe the onset and development of stuttering, as well as the production of a stuttered disruption, as the result of a dynamic and nonlinear interaction of multiple risk factors. These risk factors include genetic predisposition; speech motor abilities; and linguistic, cognitive, emotional, and environmental status. According to Smith and Kelly, the weight of each factor and how it interacts with other factors over time most likely results in considerable differences between individuals with regard to the mechanisms underlying stuttering. Therefore, stuttering results from the combined influence of multiple risk factors as opposed to having multiple causes. The clinical applicability of this model of stuttering is clear: To provide the best intervention for children and adults who stutter, we need to delineate and address the most relevant risk factors.

2. **A Behavior.** As described, stuttering as a behavior can emerge through a complex interaction of the child's overall speech and language abilities, degree of emotional arousal, length and complexity of the utterance, and degree of communicative demand in the situation at a specific point in time (proximal cause). The risk factors for either distal or proximal causes of stuttering do not need to be deficiencies in any factor

(e.g., language delay, neuromotor deficit, parental neglect). It is the interaction among factors that may lead to both the disorder and the behavior of stuttering; and the changing nature and interaction of risk factors, over time, may be responsible for the remission or persistence of stuttering.

Definitions of stuttering as a behavior describe the distinguishing characteristics of speech that are judged to represent stuttering. What does stuttered speech sound and look like to listeners? How does it differ from nonstuttered or normally fluent speech? Which behaviors of disfluent speech are not considered to be stuttering?

B. Defining the Behaviors of Stuttering

Several researchers and clinicians (e.g., Smith & Kelly, 1997) agree that different levels of definition serve different purposes; however, focus on the *behavior* of stuttering is most beneficial for treating stuttering (e.g., Wingate, 1964). This does not mean that speech-language pathologists are not interested in what may have caused a stuttering problem to emerge or what factors within and outside of the individual contribute to the persistence of stuttering. Obviously, these aspects, along with variability in the frequency and severity of stuttering across situations, provide a more complete view of the person who stutters and what factors to consider in therapy. However, speech-language pathologists, for the most part, provide treatment designed to help a client change a behavior or behaviors or to acquire new ones. To be effective, clinicians need information that will help them to define a communication disorder in terms of its relevant behavior(s). Further, the behaviors we describe as salient need to be readily observable so that we know whether the person has acquired or changed the ones of interest and whether he or she has generalized and maintained these behaviors in different contexts.

II. UNDERSTANDING THE BEHAVIOR OF STUTTERING WITHIN THE CONTEXT OF FLUENCY AND DISFLUENCY

A. What Is Speech Fluency?

During their preschool years, children simultaneously acquire the speech sounds, content, and structure of their native language. This developmental process is a dynamic one, in that these variables may not develop at the same rate. Further, articulation and language are interrelated during this period of development, such that change in one of these variables may either facilitate or depress change in the other. One example is the young child who has precocious expressive language but a phonological system that is at or slightly below age-level expectations. In this case, it may be that the child has expended a relatively large amount of cognitive resources in the acquisition of language, leaving a relatively small amount devoted to speech sound development. Further, the child's attempts to produce sophisticated language with a marginal speech motor system may lead to some disruption in output.

In addition to articulation and language, children are acquiring speech fluency during their early years. Speech fluency can be thought of as the ability to connect or link sounds, syllables, and words smoothly while speaking. Like all other aspects of speech and language, the acquisition of fluency is a developmental process that interacts in a complex way with articulation and language. In some cases, the nature of this interaction may lead to speech disfluencies in the young child.

B. What Is Speech Disfluency?

If fluent speech is characterized by smooth transitioning between speech segments, then speech disfluency (*dis* meaning "the absence of") is characterized by some disruption in easily moving to, and away from, sounds, syllables, and words. To some extent, disfluent speech is observed in the developing speech of most young children. It stands to reason that the ability to make a transition between sounds, syllables, and words smoothly both affects, and is affected by, the child's articulation and language skills. For this reason, just as children make speech and language errors while they are learning to talk, they are, to some extent, also disfluent. Disfluency, then, is a normal part of speech and language development; and as the child's articulation and language skills improve with age and time, so does the child's fluency.

With this in mind, we can appreciate the challenge of diagnosing a child to be stuttering, given that disfluent speech is an expected and relatively normal part of speech and language acquisition. When, then, is disfluent speech ever abnormal, if at all? This is where the speech-language pathologist enters the picture and determines when disfluent speech is not typical of normal speech and language development, and therefore considers the child to be stuttering. As we will see, a primary means of distinguishing stuttering from normal disfluency is to examine the qualitative differences between and among speech disfluencies.

For many years, researchers and clinicians, aware of the normal disfluency-stuttering dilemma, have sought to examine and describe the speech disfluencies produced by people judged to be normally fluent and those diagnosed to be stuttering (e.g., Conture, 1990; Johnson et al., 1959; Williams & Silverman, 1968; Williams, Silverman, & Kools, 1968). These analyses included both children and adults. The outcome of these and more recent investigations has been the development of a classification system in which disfluencies can be divided into two categories: between-word and within-word disfluencies. More recently, within-word speech disfluencies have also been referred to as stutter-like disfluencies (SLDs) (Yairi, 1997). If we consider disfluencies to reflect a disturbance in the smooth transitioning between sounds, syllables, and words, then we can think of between-word disfluencies as those in which the transitioning disruption occurs while attempting to link words together. Examples of these include phrase repetitions (e.g., "*I want, I want* to go home") and interjections (e.g., "I, **um,** want to go"). Within-word disfluencies, or SLDs, involve disruption in the smooth connection of sounds or syllables within a word. These include repetitions of sounds (e.g., "*s-s*-something for me"); repetitions of syllables (e.g., "*bu-bu*-butter and cinnamon"); repetitions of monosyllabic whole words (e.g., "**I-I-I** want a cookie"); prolongations of sounds (e.g., "*Wwww*what's your name?"); blocks (e.g., "[*silent pause*] . . . Do you want one?"); and broken words (e.g., "*G*[*silent pause*] . . . ive it to him") (adapted from Conture, 1990). Using this conceptual framework, we can describe the characteristics of different disfluencies by providing a behavioral label (e.g., sound and syllable repetition).

C. What Disfluencies Characterize Stuttering?

Over the years, numerous researchers have examined both the perceptual and the production aspects of disfluent speech. The primary questions addressed in this work have been (1) How do the speech disfluencies produced by stuttering and nonstuttering speakers differ? and (2) How do listeners perceive and judge various characteristics of disfluent speech? With regard to the second question, investigators have specifically examined the relationship between frequency (overall number), type (between and within word), and duration of speech disfluencies and the probability that listeners will judge speech to be either stuttered or not stuttered. Results from these studies have consistently shown that children and adults who stutter tend to produce a higher proportion of within-word speech disfluencies than individuals who do not stutter, and listeners are more likely to judge within-word disfluencies as being stuttered and between-word disfluencies as being not stuttered. In particular, repetitions of sounds and syllables, and to some extent, words, are the disfluency types that listeners most frequently label as stuttering. Sound prolongations are also judged to be stuttering, but less frequently than repetitions. Conversely, interjections, revisions, and phrase repetitions are most frequently considered to be not stuttered. Based on the findings from studies of production and perception, it appears that stuttering is best viewed as a relationship between speech disfluencies, listener reactions to disfluent speech, and the speaker's response to both. As such, these factors should be examined during both an evaluation and a period of diagnostic therapy in the beginning stages of treatment.

III. CONCLUSION

Stuttering can be defined and observed at different levels; all levels are important to our understanding of this complex problem. Helping people who stutter to change the behavior of stuttering, that is, the speech production behaviors that either promote fluency or interfere with the flow of speech, is the primary focus of the speech-language pathologist. Although therapy primarily focuses on changing behavior, our broader understanding of stuttering as a disorder provides important insight into the many layers associated with these behaviors. For the most part, these layers need to be examined and peeled away or replaced for behavioral changes to be maintained.

CHAPTER

2

Assessment of Stuttering

I. DIAGNOSTIC QUESTIONS DETERMINE ASSESSMENT PLANS

Stuttering intervention is a dynamic process. Dynamic means that the goals and procedures used are determined by the client's behavior and needs, and are likely to change throughout the process. A clinician typically fine-tunes the overall therapy plan to become more familiar with the client's abilities, attitudes, and concerns during the early stages of treatment. In addition, the client's family members and their issues need to be considered, and often therapy is modified to address their needs as well. Although the process of intervention should be flexible, there needs to be a starting point. Every therapeutic relationship should begin with a plan, and this plan is determined by the results of a diagnostic evaluation.

Following the evaluation, the client may be scheduled for stuttering therapy. During the initial therapy sessions, the clinician gathers in-depth information about the nature of the client's problem; the client's responsiveness to stimulation and learning style; the importance of the client's thoughts, concerns, and beliefs about the development and achievement of goals; and the amount and quality of the family's participation in the client's therapy. The clinician attempts to formulate a picture of the client and the family during this early period of diagnostic therapy. So it is helpful to consider evaluation as an ongoing process, which helps the clinician move from a somewhat pared down view of the client (i.e., Does the client stutter? If so, is therapy needed and advised?) to a more complete picture of the nature of the problem. Further, within this period of diagnostic therapy, the clinician obtains a better understanding of the client as a person with a family, who possesses certain characteristics and abilities that either promote or interfere with progress in therapy. In the following sections, we discuss the components of a fluency evaluation for both children and adults, including the significance of the various components.

A. What Are the Diagnostic Questions for Children and Adults?

When asked to evaluate a young child for stuttering, the primary questions are typically, "Is the child stuttering or at risk for stuttering?" and "Will the child experience recovery from stuttering, or will he outgrow it?" Conversely, for older, school-age children, teenagers, and adults, the main concern is not typically if the person stutters, but rather, "What is the nature of stuttering?" and "Can this person be helped?" Sometimes, children as old as nine or ten, who have been stuttering since three or four years of age, are referred because their parents or teachers are not sure whether the child's disfluency is considered normal or is stuttering. For these children, as well as for older children and adults, however, that question was answered at an earlier time. More typically these older clients want to know more about their stuttering, and the likelihood that they can obtain and benefit from therapy.

II. STUTTERING ASSESSMENT FOR CHILDREN

In this section, we outline the components of a stuttering evaluation for children. We design our assessment protocol to allow us to view the behavioral, emotional, and attitudinal aspects of stuttering, all of which make important contributions to the path that the child's stuttering will take—either a path to recovery or to a persistent stuttering problem. We start with the assumption that these three components exist in equal amounts, but with the expectation that our assessment procedures will allow us to get a sense of the

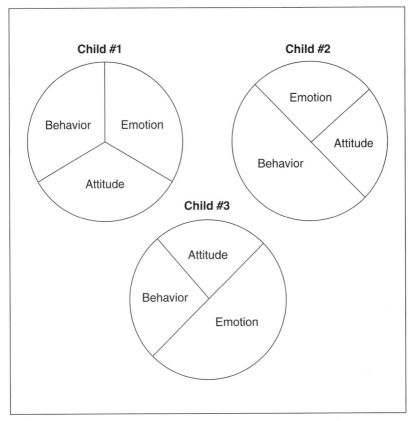

FIGURE 2.1   Hypothetical profiles weighting behavioral, emotional, and attitudinal contributions to stuttering.

relative contributions each makes to the child's stuttering. Figure 2.1 depicts three possible scenarios in which the factors are weighted differently, but obviously there are many more.

We will revisit these components in subsequent chapters, when we discuss how to set therapy agendas tailored to address the degree to which each component or factor may contribute to the child's stuttering.

Figure 2.2 (adopted from Zebrowski, 2000) shows, the diagnostic questions that need to be answered to determine whether a child stutters or is normally disfluent; the likelihood of recovery with or without therapy; and the need, desirability, and initial focus of therapy. The information required to answer these questions is provided by the objectives associated with each question.

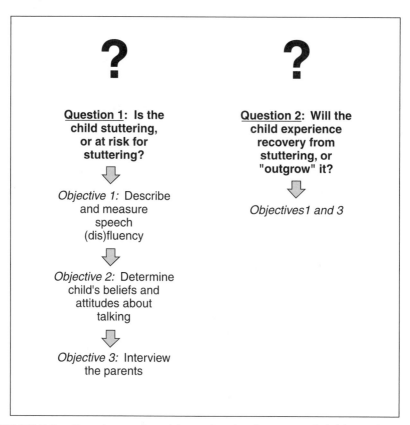

FIGURE 2.2   Questions to be addressed in the diagnosis of children who stutter. Source: Adopted from Zebrowski, 2000.

These objectives are specifically designed to uncover the behavioral (e.g., objective 1), emotional, and attitudinal (e.g., objectives 2 and 3) aspects of stuttering , as discussed earlier. The intent here is to demonstrate the data that are obtained from each evaluation objective, along with a brief interpretation of how this information helps to answer the questions.

A. Question 1: Is the Child Stuttering or at Risk for Stuttering?

1. Objective 1: Describe and Measure Speech (Dis)Fluency.

- Average frequency of speech disfluency, expressed in percent disfluent words or syllables in a predetermined number of

words, or interval of time (i.e., the percent of disfluent syllables produced in one minute of conversational speech);
- Type of speech disfluencies produced (i.e., within- and between-word disfluency), and proportion of type (in percentage) of all disfluencies produced in the sample;
- Average duration or length of 10 to 20 instances of speech disfluency;
- Presence or absence of associated (or secondary) behaviors;
- Severity of disfluency, judged as mild, moderate, or severe;
- Average speech rate, expressed as the number of words or syllables per minute or second;
- Evaluation of phonological and language status; and
- Evaluation of oral mechanism structure and function.

2. **Interpretation of the Results from Objective 1.**

   a. Average Frequency of Speech Disfluency. The frequency of speech disfluency provides a measure of the extent to which disfluent productions are likely to be hampering the child's communication in comparison with his peers. Obviously, the higher the frequency of disfluency, regardless of type, the more likely it will be that listeners will judge the child's speech to be abnormal to some degree. Further, a fairly high frequency of disfluency increases the probability that the child will experience incomplete or failed attempts at oral communication and expression.

   In a review of studies conducted through 1997, Yairi (1997) concluded that preschool-age children who stutter produce an average of 17 speech disfluencies of all types in 100 syllables of speech. Slightly higher levels of 19 to 20 disfluencies per 100 syllables were found for children closer to the onset of stuttering. In contrast, preschool-age children who do not stutter produce an average of 6 to 8 disfluencies in 100 syllables (Yairi, 1997). Due to averages, a particular child may produce slightly more or fewer disfluencies than the mean.

   b. Type of Speech Disfluency and Proportion of Type. In addition to producing more disfluencies overall, research has consistently shown that children ultimately diagnosed to be stuttering, regardless of age, produce more within-word, or stutterlike disfluencies (SLD; sound/syllable repetitions and sound prolongations) than children of normal fluency. Specifically as a group, preschool children who stutter produce a *minimum* of three to four within-word or stutterlike disfluencies per 100 syllables (Yairi, 1997), while their nonstuttering peers typically produce fewer than three stutterlike disfluencies per 100 syllables. Further, when viewed as a proportion of the total number of disfluencies produced overall, the percentage of SLDs produced by nonstuttering children "is always under 50% and is most nearly near 35%" (Yairi, 1997, p. 58). In contrast, an average of 65% or more SLDs has been found in the speech of preschool children who stutter, nearly twice that for children who do not stutter (Ambrose & Yairi, 1999). Finally, young children who stutter have been observed to produce "clustered" disfluencies, which are productions of two or more stutterlike or within-word disfluencies "on adjacent sounds, syllables or words within an utterance" (Conture, 1997, p. 250). These children tend to produce clusters in which there are two stutterlike elements about 32% of the time, while their fluent peers have not been observed to produce clustered disfluencies at all (LaSalle & Conture, 1995).

Given these data, we use the rather conservative judgment rule that children who produce at least three within-word or clustered disfluencies in 100 syllables of conversational speech are considered to be stuttering or at risk for developing stuttering. The higher the proportion of within-word disfluencies in the total number of speech disfluencies produced (which is usually the case), the more likely it will be that listeners will judge the child to be stuttering. One additional clinical note: Oftentimes the proportions of different disfluency types change as a result of the natural recovery process (e.g., fewer within-word disfluencies over time, beginning with stuttering onset), as a result of treatment, or as the child's stuttering persists and becomes chronic. Therefore, type and proportion of type across time can be indicative of change, in either a positive or negative direction.

c. Average Duration of Speech Disfluency. Duration, particularly of within-word disfluencies, is another measure of the extent to which disfluent production is affecting the child's output and communicative success. Further, duration can provide some indication of the amount of difficulty the child is experiencing when attempting to smoothly transition between sounds, syllables, and words. Studies have shown that as a group, children who stutter tend to produce sound/syllable repetitions and sound prolongations averaging 0.50 to 0.75 sec in duration. The range of durations is from 0.25 sec or less, to 1 sec and longer. It is not unusual for young children to produce stuttered disruptions which are 0.25 sec or shorter. Such disruptions are extremely difficult, if not impossible, to measure with a handheld stopwatch. We refer to the duration of these brief, difficult-to-measure disfluencies as "reaction time disruptions," which is roughly the amount of time it takes one to push down and release the button on a stop watch. Similar to proportion of type, duration often changes as a result of treatment. The child's increased ability to move smoothly into and away from syllables and words is reflected in stuttered disruptions of decreasing length over time.

Comparisons of children who do and do not stutter for overall duration of within-word or stutterlike disfluencies have yielded tremendous overlap, with no clear criteria for differentiating the two groups. In fact, preschool children who stutter may produce shorter durations of sound/syllable repetitions and sound prolongations. Recent data suggest that this may be due to the observation that young children who stutter produce shorter pauses between repeated units within repetitions of sounds, syllables, and monosyllabic words. Note that this difference is only apparent in preschoolers.

d. Associated Behaviors. Sometimes referred to as secondary behaviors, associated behaviors are thought to be related to the child's developing awareness, that he or she is experiencing some difficulty talking (at least) or is stuttering (at most). These actions can take many forms such as head, torso, or limb movement; audible inhalations or exhalations; and visible muscular tension in the orofacial muscles. In young children, however, the most frequently observed associated behaviors involve the eyes. Some of the more common eye behaviors include closing, blinking, or squeezing the eyes shut during moments of stuttering, lateral or vertical eye movement, and consistent loss of eye contact during stuttered disruptions. In many cases, these rather subtle eye behaviors are relatively difficult to observe especially when they accompany

very short, or fleeting, disfluencies. Of diagnostic significance is that children as close to stuttering onset as one
month have been shown to display associated behaviors.
Children who are normally disfluent do not exhibit associated behaviors with their disfluent productions. The presence
of associated behaviors suggests that the child's awareness
might motivate him or her to produce behaviors intended to
"keep from stuttering." Over time, these behaviors (e.g., using inappropriately high amounts of laryngeal tension when
disfluent) are likely to become a part of the chronic stuttering
pattern.

e. Severity of Stuttering. Severity of stuttering is a global
judgment based on listeners' perceptions of the frequency,
type, and duration of disfluent speech, as well as the presence or absence of associated behaviors. It is helpful in that
it gives clinicians a common language to describe the general character of a child's stuttering problem (i.e., mild,
moderate, severe), but it is not very useful in describing the
behaviors of stuttering produced by individual children.
Further, while studies have shown some degree of reliabil-
ity in making judgments of stuttering severity, listeners vary
with regard to their decisions about severity. The conven-
tional way of determining stuttering severity is to rank the
individual's speech on a scale, where the low end reflects
"no stuttering" and the high end reflects "very severe stuttering." The *Scale for Rating the Severity of Stuttering*
(Johnson, Darley, & Spriestersbach, 1963) is one such tool,
and the *Stuttering Severity Instrument for Children and
Adults—3* (SSI-3) (Riley, 1994) is another. The first allows
a clinician to assign an overall severity rating from 0 to 7,
while the latter uses a composite score based on independent judgments or measures of frequency, duration, and associated behaviors to yield a rating of severity (e.g., mild,
moderate). In addition to these instruments, *Stuttering
Prediction Instrument for Young Children* (SPI) (Riley,
1981) provides clinicians with a set of interview questions
for the parents and measures to obtain from the child's
speech (similar to those described for objective 1). The SPI
allows the clinician to use data collected from both the parent and the child to predict the probability that the child will
develop chronic stuttering.

f. Speech Rate. Speech rate is a valuable measure in that it completes the overall picture, showing the impact that disfluency or stuttering has on speech output. The speaking rate measure that best shows this effect is overall rate, which takes into consideration all of the within-utterance pauses and disfluencies when calculated. In this case, it follows that there is an inverse relationship between frequency and duration of pauses/disfluencies and speech rate; that is, the longer and/or more frequent these disruptions, the fewer the words (or syllables) produced per unit time. So, if the average overall speech rate for 4-year-old children is 153 words per minute (e.g., Kelly & Conture, 1992), then a same-age child whose stuttering consists of a relatively high frequency of disfluencies averaging 0.5 sec, may produce fewer words in a minute's time. This mismatch in output may put some children who stutter at a considerable disadvantage in conversational exchanges with their peers, and at even more of a disadvantage when talking with adults, whose typical rate may be 200 words per minute or more. Finally, similar to frequency, type, and duration of stuttering, speaking rate changes as a result of therapy. The more fluently a child speaks, and/or the shorter the duration of those disfluencies, the more syllables or words per unit time the child can produce. The significance here is that the communication "playing field" is leveled, so that the child is more likely to be an equal participant in verbal exchanges.

3. **Objective 2: Determine Child's Beliefs and Attitudes about Talking.** It is important to "talk about talking" with children who are developmentally able and willing to do so. The purpose is to determine the following:

   • Child's level of awareness about what stuttering is
   • Child's thoughts and beliefs about why he or she stutters
   • Child's awareness of anything he or she does to help
   • Child's level of distress or worry
   • Child's perception of the parents' level of distress or worry

   Following are possible questions to ask the child in order to obtain this information.

   • Do you know why you came to see me today?
   • Is talking easy for you, or is it hard? Is it easy sometimes and hard at other times? When is it easy, and when is it hard?

- Why do you think that talking is hard for you sometimes?
- What do you do when it's hard to talk? What does it sound like?
- Do you like to talk?
- How worried are you about talking? How worried are your parents about your talking? (Ask the child to rate on a scale, with 1 being "not worried at all," and 7 being "the most worried.")

An additional way to assess the child's attitudes about speaking is through the *Children's Attitudes about Talking* (Brutten and Dunham 1989), which allows the clinician to compare responses of a child who stutters to a series of true/false statements about talking, with those obtained from nonstuttering children across a range of ages. This questionnaire was administered to Belgian children who did and did not stutter, and the authors observed that as a group, the stuttering children showed an increase in speech-associated *negative* attitudes with age, while the normally fluent children displayed an increase in *positive* attitudes about talking with age.

4. **Interpretation of the Results from Objective 2.** As we will discuss later in this book, stuttering therapy for children can take either a direct or an indirect approach (Conture, 1990). Although a number of factors guide the decision about which is best (e.g., child's age, cognitive and language abilities), an important one is the degree to which the child is negatively reacting to the stuttering. In most cases, it is unlikely that preschoolers have developed any pervasive feelings or attitudes about their stuttering, but school-age children who stutter typically are aware and possibly concerned about their disfluent speech. If awareness of stuttering is present, it is more likely that a child is having thoughts that something is different about the way they talk and/or showing signs that talking is hard for them.

An additional factor is the degree to which children try to help themselves talk more easily. Some children may react by abandoning what they are saying, asking significant others about their difficulties (e.g., "Mommy, why can't I talk?"), or using excessive muscular tension, stopping, or pushing out air in an attempt to "get the word out." These thoughts and reactions may be influenced by the child's own temperament (Guitar, 1998) as well as the reactions of significant others (e.g., parents) to the child and to the stuttering. There is no current evidence to suggest children who react to their own stuttering in these ways are more likely to continue to stutter. Many theorists and clinicians, however, have discussed the potential influence of learning processes on the development of escape and avoidance behaviors that may reinforce, exacerbate, and potentially maintain stuttering over time (Starkweather, 1997; Starkweather, Gottwald, & Halfond, 1990).

In cases when the child is aware and reacting negatively to stuttering, intervention is warranted and some direct attention needs to be paid to the child's perceptions and emotional reactions. For young children, this usually takes the form of brief, but consistent intervals of gentle questioning and listening, followed by general reassurance that it is okay to stutter, and that the clinician is there to help. Clinical interventions with young children who stutter include parent counseling, clinician modeling, and direct and indirect therapy.

5. **Objective 3: Interview the Parents.** The purpose of the parent interview is to obtain the standard case history information regarding the child's developmental, medical, social, and educational history, as well as the history and development of the stuttering problem. It is also important to ask about the family history of stuttering or other communication or learning problems. Finally, the interview should be used to determine the questions, beliefs, and concerns the parents have about stuttering and their child. Specific questions include the following:

   • When was the problem first noticed? How old was the child?
   • Who first noticed the problem? What did that person do?
   • What was the child's speech like when the problem was first noticed? Show me what disfluencies looked and sounded like.
   • What is the child's speech like now? How has it changed since the problem first started?
   • Has the frequency and type of disfluency changed over time? Do you observe fairly consistent amounts of disfluency from day to day and week to week, or does this seem to vary?
   • Is there a history of stuttering in either the paternal or maternal family? Who? Did affected family members "recover" or "outgrow" stuttering? When (e.g., soon after onset, during childhood, after therapy)?
   • What do you and other family members do when the child stutters? Why do you do this? Does it help?

- Have others commented about your child's speech? What have they said?
- Why do you think your child stutters (or is disfluent)? What do you think causes stuttering?
- What are your primary concerns about your child at this time? What would you like to obtain from this evaluation?

6. **Interpretation of the Results from Objective 3.** The information you obtain from the parent interview is key to answering the second diagnostic question: Will the child experience recovery from stuttering? We will discuss the interpretation of the necessary information in the next section. In addition to providing information that helps predict unassisted recovery, the parents' responses to interview questions provide some direction toward intervention. For example, if the parents report that they routinely provide the child with instructions on how to talk either during or after the child's disfluencies, then you will want to find out what the parents say. Parental comments such as, "Slow down and think about what you want to say" or "Take a deep breath" may not be harmful, but they are not likely to help and might indicate to the child that his or her speech is a problem that the parents want to stop. Similarly, the beliefs and attitudes about stuttering and child development that the parents exhibit frequently provide issues for family counseling. For example, parents who believe that something they either did or failed to do somehow caused the child's stuttering need information about the role of the child's environment in the onset and development of stuttering. Specifically, in these cases parents need to understand that stuttering most likely emerges from a complex interaction between multiple risk factors, and that the interplay between and among these risk factors is likely to be different for individual children.

Related to this is an understanding of the important difference between causal as opposed to contributing variables. In addition, parents who express feelings of guilt relating to the child's stuttering will require counseling to manage these and related emotions. Finally, as with all parent interviews, the clinician will obtain information that will help to determine any additional areas for later evaluation (e.g., language, cognition), and issues that might affect therapy, such as previous diagnoses of attention deficit disorder (ADD), emotional or health problems, and family problems.

B. Question 2: Will the Child Experience Recovery from Stuttering, or "Outgrow" It?

1. **Interpretation of the Results from Objectives 1 and 3.** Once you have answered the first diagnostic question, you will need to address the second question about spontaneous or unassisted recovery. Unassisted recovery refers to the remission of stuttering without formal intervention. Unfortunately, there is no definitive answer to this question; however, in recent years Yairi and his colleagues at the University of Illinois (Champaign) have made insightful observations into the problem of predicting which children will recover from stuttering and which will not (e.g., Paden, Yairi, & Ambrose, 1999; Watkins, Yairi, & Ambrose, 1999; Yairi & Ambrose, 1999). These researchers followed a large group of young children who were close to the onset of stuttering, with the purpose of describing patterns of stuttering development. Over the course of the study, they observed that a large proportion of children recovered. This phenomenon allowed Yairi and his associates to analyze their data with an eye toward identifying specific factors that were related to either the remission or perpetuation of stuttering. Among others, these factors included the child's age at onset; the length of time the child has been stuttering (also referred to as the post-onset interval); family history of stuttering; recovery or persistence patterns of affected family members; gender; the decline, increase, or stability of sound/syllable and word repetitions over time; and the presence of coexisting problems.

Using the results from these and earlier studies, we can evaluate the information obtained through objectives 1 and 3 to answer this second question. That is, we use observations made while assessing the child's speech, and information provided by the parents, to make a well-informed prediction of the probability of recovery. The parents must clearly understand that there is no variable or combination of variables that conclusively points to recovery from stuttering (or the continued development of stuttering); however, the previously discussed research findings allow us to speculate about the likelihood of recovery for particular children.

In general, approximately 74% of young children who are diagnosed to be stuttering will experience unassisted recovery. Children who recover from stuttering do so relatively soon after the problem is first noted, usually within 6 to 36 months post onset. The probability of unassisted recovery increases with the presence of each of the following factors: female gender, stuttering onset prior to age three, a negative family history of stuttering *or* a positive family history where the affected family member recovered in childhood, observations of speech indicate an immediate and steady decline in the frequency of sound/syllable and word repetitions and sound prolongations over time, and no concomitant speech or language problems.

2. **After the Diagnosis: Fine-Tuning for the Treatment Plan.** After completing the evaluation objectives interpretation of results and formulating the preliminary decisions about treatment (e.g., what general approach to take, how often to schedule therapy, amount and type of family participation in therapy), it is important to engage in a relatively brief fine-tuning of the treatment plan. During this interval of "diagnostic therapy," the clinician obtains a more comprehensive view of the child and family through a combination of observation and further evaluation. Factors to examine during this phase of treatment include the following:

   a. Variability of Stuttering Frequency. During the initial period of diagnostic therapy, the clinician should assess the degree of variability in the frequency of stuttering across different contexts. It is important to recognize that for childhood stuttering, variability is normal, not only in the frequency of disfluency, but also in the duration and type of stuttering behavior. It is important to note, too, that in many cases the speech sample(s) collected during the diagnostic evaluation are sufficient to allow us to make the diagnosis of stuttering, but are too limited to allow us to assess the "plasticity" of the problem. That is, does the child produce roughly the same frequency, duration, and type of stuttering from situation to situation and day to day; or are there situations and times in which the child is essentially fluent, followed closely by those during which it seems as though every other word is stuttered? Although usually more exasperating for parents, the second scenario is more typical of early stuttering, which is likely to resolve. The first scenario is more representative of chronic stuttering which is not likely to show remission without intervention. Yairi and his colleagues have shown that young children close to stuttering onset, who show unassisted recovery from stuttering, exhibit consistent reductions in the frequency of stutteringlike disfluencies (i.e., sound/syllable and whole-word repetitions and sound prolongations) almost immediately post onset, whereas those children whose stuttering persists do not demonstrate such reductions. Further, studies have shown that for some children, the frequency of stuttering is higher at home as opposed to in the clinic, and is also highly variable from day to day within the same context. These are important reasons to collect speech samples across different in- and out-of-clinic situations and settings, and across time (Ingham & Riley, 1998).

b. Temporal Aspects of Parent-Child Conversation. It is well known that conversational partners tend to become attuned to certain aspects of speech while talking with one another. In particular, such behaviors as speaking rate, duration of turn-switching pauses, number and duration of pauses within individual turns, and length of turns become correlated during conversation. Further, there is mutual influence in the development of this attunement or conversational congruence; that is, the two speakers affect each other in a bidirectional manner. This phenomenon has been observed in studies of young children who are talking with their parents.

Given this phenomenon, it seems reasonable to speculate that the tempo or timing rhythm of the parent-child conversation may be affected by the child's stuttering. In these cases, parents may be more inclined to interrupt the child or engage in simultaneous talking as an attempt to repair the conversational rhythm, trying to bring it back to normal. In turn, the child may interrupt or talk simultaneously in order to hold the floor or complement the parents' behavior in some way.

To assess the potentially stressful effects of this temporal incongruity, the clinician should note the parents' speech rate and turn-taking behaviors as compared with the child's in conversation. A difference between the child's rate and the parents' rate (dyadic rate) exceeding 100 syllables per minute (Kelly & Conture, 1992) suggests an imbalance of output between the child and the parents that might be in some way stressful for the child. For example, in this situation the child may experience subtle, but chronic pressure to keep up with the tempo of the conversation. In turn, this experience may lead to a general feeling of time urgency for the child, which is a feeling of being rushed to verbally communicate. Although neither the relationship between parent-child speech rates nor the speech rates of either parents or children alone have been shown to cause stuttering, it is known that a general slowing of overall speech rate and increased duration of turn-switching pauses facilitates fluency for some children. It may be the case that certain aspects of parent-child interaction need to be modified through parental counseling and modeling to increase the probability that the child will produce fluent speech.

c. Child's Language and Phonological Status. Certain evidence indicates some children who stutter exhibit concomitant problems in language and phonological development. Of the two, there appears to be a higher incidence of phonological deficit in young children who stutter as a group (Paden & Yairi, 1996). More recent work by Paden et al. (1999) indicates that phonological delay or a slow-developing phonological system is predictive of persistent stuttering in children at or close to stuttering onset. In a related study, Watkins et al. (1999) showed that 2- to 3-year-old children who were just beginning to stutter displayed asynchronies in their language and phonological abilities, such that phonology was at or slightly below age-level expectations and language skills were well above. They concluded that some children who stutter (notably the youngest), may experience "developmental trade-offs" (p. 1133), whereby the resources required for precocious or advanced abilities in one area of development (e.g., expressive language) comes at a cost to another area (e.g., fluency or phonological abilities). This makes sense from a resource allocation perspective; that is, unequal distribution of a finite amount of resources requires that some areas of development receive a smaller proportion of the available cognitive resources than others.

Whatever the case, it is important to assess the language and phonological status of children who stutter during the period of diagnostic therapy. In addition to the identification of relative strengths and needs, it is important to evaluate such dimensions as the relationship between stuttering and language complexity, demand or function, the location or "loci" of stuttering within utterances, and the development of potential fluency "stressors" such as a large discrepancy between phonological and language abilities. Further, a thorough assessment of the child's language and phonological abilities allows the clinician to consider what aspects of the child's speech and language are most responsible for compromised communication. For example, is the child's intelligibility more of a hindrance to communication than his or her stuttering? Is a limited vocabulary and relatively small mean length of utterance more problematic than the handful of speech-sound errors and rather easily produced disfluencies? Or are several concomitant problems weighted about equally? Sorting out these issues is critical when prioritizing treatment goals and objectives, and the information required to do so is often not sought or readily observable given the time constraints of a standard diagnostic evaluation.

d. Topic Contextualization. Some evidence shows that children produce more and more fluent language when the topic of conversation is contextualized, meaning that the topic is familiar, meaningful, or interesting to the child, and there are auditory or visual "props" related to the topic to assist the child in language formulation (Smith, 1999). On the other hand, additional work has shown just the opposite. That is, children produce longer and more complex utterances and more fluent speech when topics are highly decontextualized, meaning children talk about things that are not in the "here and now" without the aid of contextual support (Masterson & Kamhi, 1991). Both observations seem reasonable. The observation that increased contextualization yields more fluency makes sense in that it suggests that fluency is aided by a reduced demand for ideational formulation. The idea that more contextualization yields less fluency also makes sense if one agrees that decontextualized topics tend to make the speaker more sensitive to listener needs and perhaps more thorough and careful when providing information. It is likely that different children who stutter will respond in idiosyncratic ways to changes in contextualization. That being the case, during the period of diagnostic therapy, the clinician should look at the affects of changes in amount and type of topic contextualization and the child's degree of speech fluency. Doing so will provide a direction for development of the speech stimuli used in treatment.

e. Hierarchy of Speaking Situations. Similar to the relationship between language complexity and stuttering, for many children who stutter there is a relationship between specific speaking situations and stuttering. While such a relationship is more likely for children and adults with persistent stuttering problems, even young children who have been stuttering for a relatively short time can come to equate certain communicative acts or situations with stuttering and others with fluency. This typical phenomenon in the development of chronic stuttering is often one of the most difficult aspects of the problem, because when children come to expect or anticipate that they will stutter in a particular situation, they will react to this feeling of anticipation by trying to keep from stuttering. This "trying not to" (Williams, 1979) behavior usually involves some form of physical struggle or interference, such as breath holding, turning off the voice, or making physically tense and fixated articulatory postures. Johnson and others (1959) state that stuttering becomes the things the child does to avoid stuttering.

To gain a sense of what situations the child may associate with stuttering (and thus "trying not to"), it is helpful to devote a portion of diagnostic therapy to the construction of a situational hierarchy. In doing so, the clinician helps the child to think of speaking situations that are the most likely to be associated with stuttering, as well as those that are the least associated with stuttering (or the most likely to be related to fluency). These situations can include places, people, specific topics or expression (e.g., saying one's name or saying a problem word), and so on. Constructing a hierarchy provides the child and the clinician with a good opportunity to discuss issues associated with stuttering, and in that way conveys the message that it is okay to talk about stuttering. In addition, this task requires children to analyze their stuttering in a fairly objective way, and for many children is the first step in separating stuttering from self. Once the hierarchy has been constructed using terms the child understands (e.g., "hard-to-easy," "most stuttering-to-least stuttering"), the clinician can help the child to practice newly learned speech strategies in either simulated or real situations on the hierarchy starting with the easiest and progressing slowly to the most difficult. For very young children, the hierarchy they create will most likely have only a few situations because of their limited experience. For older children, however, especially those who might be sensitive to the environment, these situational hierarchies can contain a variety of situations that seem to differ only slightly. In these cases, hierarchy construction can be a time-consuming production, but it is well worth the effort.

III. STUTTERING ASSESSMENT IN ADULTS

As described earlier, for adults the primary questions in a stuttering evaluation are "What is the nature of stuttering?" and "Will treatment help?" The overwhelming majority of adults who stutter have been doing so since they were preschoolers, and the diagnosis of stuttering was made at some point in their childhood. When these adults come to the clinic for an evaluation, it is usually because they are interested in exploring therapy options and want to know what is available. Most of these clients have a history of therapy, and for some, therapy has been sporadic over many years. Some may have never received any treatment for their stuttering. Whatever the case, the clinician needs to obtain enough information to gain an understanding of (1) the nature of the person's stuttering behavior, including the frequency, type, duration, and variability; (2) the individual's beliefs and attitudes about talking and stuttering; and (3) any feelings or concerns the individual has about people who stutter.

Similar to Figure 2.2, Figure 2.3 (Zebrowski, 2000) provides a schematic representation of the three primary questions for the assessment of stuttering in adults, and the assessment objectives for answering these questions. Our assessment questions for adults who stutter differ from those we ask when appraising children. For adults, the initial question is, "What is the nature of the disfluent speech?" The second and third questions relate to therapy: "Is therapy warranted as well as recommended? If so, what should be the focus of therapy?"

A. Question 1: What Is the Nature of the Disfluent Speech?

1. **Objective 1: Describe and Measure Speech (Dis)Fluency.** For the clinician to develop an in-depth view of the characteristics of the client's stuttered and fluent speech, the clinician will have to obtain the same basic measures as described earlier for children. That is, the clinician needs to measure the average frequency of disfluency, the types of different disfluencies produced and the proportion of different types, the average duration of stuttered disruptions, the presence or absence of associated behaviors, the overall severity of the problem, the average speech rate in conversational speech,

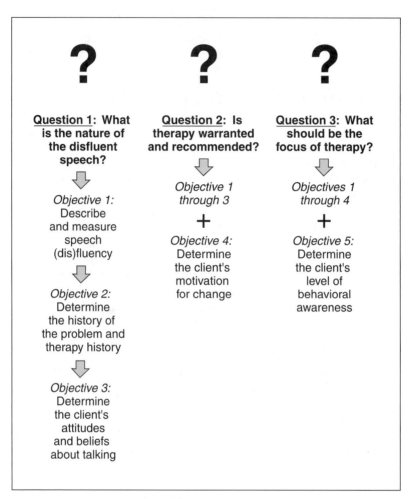

FIGURE 2.3   Questions to be addressed in the diagnosis of adults who stutter.

and the structure and function of the oral mechanism from one or multiple speech samples.

This behavioral information will help the clinician and the client to compare the client's stuttered speech with his or her own non-stuttering or normally fluent speech, and in doing so will provide direction for treatment goals. A helpful structure for this type of analytical observation was provided by Adams (1974), and involves using the processes associated with fluent speech production as reference points against which to compare stuttered speech. The main idea is that the clinician needs to be able to speculate about what the client does to produce stuttered or disfluent speech, and how that behavioral pattern differs from what he or she does to produce smooth, fluent speech. Together with the client, treatment strategies are then developed to help identify not only when stuttering occurs, but also what the client does to interfere with the flow of speech.

For example, suppose the client produces a high proportion of inaudible sound prolongations at the beginning of utterances. The clinician notes that the client seems to be holding or "freezing" his speech articulators, while simultaneously holding his breath and halting phonation. Since smooth, fluent speech requires airflow, voicing, and continuous movement of the speech articulators, it is apparent that the client needs to learn how to initiate or maintain these behaviors at those points in the speech stream where he is aware of disrupting them (or is beginning to disrupt them).

2. **Objective 2: Determine the History of the Problem and Therapy History.** During the intake interview, the clinician needs to obtain a history of the stuttering problem, along with a history of the treatment the client has obtained. It is especially important to know the amount, type, and effectiveness of any past therapy. The adult client may have received stuttering treatment in the past, typically at school. For many clients, therapy during elementary or junior high is the most recent treatment they received prior to the present referral. They usually have experienced some progress at that time, but no long-term maintenance. As adults, concerns about stuttering may have taken a backseat to other life issues, and they may be contemplating a return to therapy again. The motivation to explore therapy options is often brought about by some change or changes in the individual's life. For example, a new job or the desire to change jobs, new job responsibilities, a new significant other or partner, a new child, or a general sense that the time is right to concentrate on speech. In other cases, the client has a very long history of therapy, and has been consistently enrolled in treatment for several years, but has made limited progress. Whatever the situation, the clinician

should ask the following questions to gain perspective on where the client is in the treatment process.

- Have you received treatment for stuttering?
- When, how much, and where? (The clinician should obtain specific information about the number and duration of therapy intervals.)
- What were the strategies or concepts taught?
- How effective was therapy?
- If not effective, why not?
- What kinds of things do you think you need right now to help you?
- What are your expectations now for therapy?

The clinician should attend to clients' openness about their stuttering and therapy history. If clients do not or cannot talk candidly about their stuttering and treatment experiences, then it is less likely that they will be able to actively participate in the therapy process, at least initially. The clinician needs to be able to gauge how involved clients will be in the early stages of treatment and the potential for a genuine commitment to the treatment objectives. A key therapy goal is that clients eventually become their own clinician, and the likelihood that this goal will be met is high if they are willing and able, with the clinician's help, to assess objectively their behaviors, attitudes, specifics, and importance of the stuttering therapy experiences.

3. **Objective 3: Determine the Client's Attitudes and Beliefs about Talking.** During the intake interview, the clinician must attempt to uncover not only client attitudes about stuttering, but also beliefs about talking and stuttering. Through interview questions and written questionnaires, it is possible to obtain an understanding of the client's perspectives on stuttering and how the client views himself or herself as someone who stutters. As Williams (1979) pointed out, although there are as many unique ideas and beliefs about stuttering as there are people who stutter, some common ones may get in the way of treatment progress. For example, if clients believe that stuttering is something that "just happens" or is something that they "have" because of who they are, then it stands to reason that those beliefs will interfere with learning to change stuttering behavior. When the focus of control is external to the individual, this engenders a belief that nothing can be done to change a behavior. Given that stuttering therapy is largely behavioral, it is easy to see how this attitude may under-

mine clients' beliefs and confidence in their ability to change, and the clinician's ability to facilitate such change.

In addition to attitudes and beliefs about the nature of stuttering and its causality, it is important to assess the client's attitudes about communication and stuttering. In other words, does the fact that the client stutters affect decisions about talking with others? Does the client avoid certain topics, speaking situations, people, events, and so forth, because of concerns about stuttering? Does the anticipation of stuttering prevent the client from participating in certain activities or conversations, or from entering specific careers? Does the client possess beliefs about what participation in therapy might imply to friends and associates? We experienced this first-hand when we observed that one of our clients, a young college-age man, was unwilling or unable to practice any of the strategies he had successfully learned in therapy while talking with anyone his own age in everyday conversation. He was very successful in the therapy room, in the clinic building, and elsewhere in structured tasks. When it came time to practice in "real life," he refused. Finally, after probing, the client admitted that he was concerned that friends and acquaintances would notice if he used "smooth speech," or if he moved through a moment of stuttering using one of the strategies he had learned. He expressed the belief that if his attempts to change his speech were evident to his listeners on some level, they would interpret this as an indication that his stuttering bothered him to such an extent that he was doing something about it. The stuttering did not concern him, not the significant extent to which stuttering compromised his communication, but rather the fact that others would think he was bothered by his stuttering. This example shows how beliefs can hinder progress.

Besides asking the client questions about beliefs and attitudes, the clinician can administer such questionnaires as the Erickson Scale of Communication Attitude (Andrews & Cutler, 1974; modified version), which contains a series of statements about communication that the client can personally indicate as being either true or false. Norms are available for both stuttering and non-stuttering adults.

Whatever the case, the client's attitudes, beliefs, and feelings about stuttering can often negatively influence personal confidence in the clinician's ability to help. For some clients, the early stages of stuttering treatment will need to include reevaluation and modification of attitudes and beliefs about stuttering before any benefit can be gained from treatment.

B. Question 2: Is Therapy Warranted and Recommended?

1. Objective 4: Determine the Client's Motivation for Change. After obtaining enough information to answer the first question, the clinician must decide whether treatment is warranted and whether it will be recommended. Note that for various reasons, a speech-language pathologist might not recommend therapy at a certain time, even though it is evident that the client will not improve speech fluency without intervention. To decide whether to recommend treatment now or at a later date, the clinician needs to consider the information obtained during the speech evaluation, the client's attitudes and beliefs about stuttering (objective 3), and a related issue, the client's motivation for change (objective 4).

Any type of behavioral intervention, including therapy for stuttering, requires the client's active participation. A high level of involvement in self-change usually stems from the combination of (1) a strong desire to change, (2) belief that one can do what it takes to make changes, (3) the ability to devote time and attention to the change process, and (4) patience and resilience. It is difficult, at best, for the clinician to know whether the adult who stutters possesses all of these attributes after one or two diagnostic sessions. Usually the client's level of motivation becomes more evident as the clinician-client relationship develops.

It is possible, however, to gain some beginning insight into the client's motivation for seeking help during the diagnostic process. During the intake interview, the clinician should ask the client why he has come for an evaluation at this point in time. The overwhelming majority of adults who stutter have been doing so since the preschool years; it is possible that they had a number of opportunities to receive stuttering therapy over the years, but for some reason they did not. Thus, the clinician needs to gain an understanding of what is motivating the client to seek professional help *now*. What are the life circumstances that resulted in the referral? How do these circumstances relate to the client's motivation to change?

Perhaps the best-case scenario is when the client decides that he or she is unwilling to struggle with stuttering any further. In these cases, the issue is that the person is tired of working so hard to hide the stuttering. At any rate, the primary motivation is personal desire for change, not because a spouse, partner, friend, or employer wants the change, not because a job or a job promotion depends on speaking more fluently (although this certainly happens), and not because a life change looms in the near future (e.g., college graduation) and the client wants to "fix" the stuttering before the event. Clients who are motivated to change their speech for themselves, rather than for another person, or because stuttering will prevent them from attaining a career or personal goal, may be more likely to remain motivated for the long road ahead in therapy (Zebrowski, 2000).

C. Question 3: What Should Be the Focus of Therapy?

If the diagnostic findings lead the clinician to decide that therapy is both recommended and warranted, then it is important to make one or two initial suggestions for therapy focus at the time of the evaluation. These suggestions should be primarily geared toward the initial stages of therapy; in other words, it is difficult to design an entire treatment plan before commencing with therapy, as both the client's reaction to therapy and his or her general needs will evolve over time. However, it is important to generate some preliminary ideas for the initial focus of therapy.

In some cases, the client may require a good deal of education about stuttering in general, and his or her own stuttering specifically. The client may need to obtain some additional counseling for issues related to stuttering, or for some that may not be directly related, but that impose obstacles to therapy participation. The clinician will use all of the information in objectives 1 through 4 to make these initial therapy recommendations, along with the observations made while attempting to achieve objective 5.

1. **Objective 5: Determine the Client's Level of Behavioral Awareness.** Having behavioral awareness means having the ability to *feel* different modes of speech and to contrast them. Feeling the change as a person moves from one speech mode to another, while changing or transitioning, is also an important aspect of the behavioral awareness necessary for fluency. In stuttering treatment, the two production modes of interest are fluent speech and stuttered speech. Applying either a stuttering modification or integrated

approach, the client will need to be aware of *what* he does to produce both fluent and stuttered speech, and *when* he is producing either. It is helpful to gather some observations about the client's level of behavioral awareness during the evaluation before developing a treatment plan.

One good method involves using a strategy that Conture (1990) has described as "on-line" identification. This skill is typically taught as a part of the treatment plan, and usually takes some time and practice to develop. By asking clients to identify instances of their own stuttering during the evaluation, however, the clinician can gauge the amount of time and attention that will need to be devoted to this skill in therapy. It is relatively easy to do this during evaluations. Toward the end of the assessment session, the clinician asks clients to read from a short passage or briefly describe a picture, and either raise a finger or tap the table as soon as they *feel* themselves beginning to use stuttered speech (or to "interfere"). It is important to distinguish between hearing, seeing, and feeling these interferences. To make speech changes, clients need to know *when* they are stuttering, and *what* they are doing at that time; thus, clients must be tuned in to the physical feeling of speech. Some clients will identify (i.e., raise a finger) their stuttering *after* they have produced them, some will identify *during,* some *before,* and some not at all, or will refuse to attempt the task. Whatever the client does in response to the clinician's request to identify stuttering provides useful information for subsequent therapy. For example, if the client accurately identifies stuttering after producing a stuttered disruption, this suggests that therapy should focus on speeding up the identification process. If the client refuses to participate in the task, it indicates that he is not ready to confront stuttering, perhaps at all or maybe just his own. In this case, early therapy might need to focus on desensitization and perhaps some "off-line" identification strategies (identifying fluent, disfluent, and stuttered speech in the speech of others, from audio or videotaped samples) before moving to self-identification.

IV. CONCLUSION

Stuttering intervention is a dynamic process that begins with a diagnostic evaluation. This initial assessment becomes the starting point for the therapeutic relationship and provides the foundation for the treatment plan. It is helpful to structure the assessment around a series of questions that need to be answered and to develop methods that will obtain the information necessary to do so. The diagnostic questions for children and adults will naturally be different in some respects. For example, the primary diagnostic question for children concerns the distinction between stuttering and normal disfluency. Is the child stuttering or at risk for stuttering? To answer this fundamental question, the clinician needs to obtain relevant background information from the parents and analyze the child's speech fluency in very specific ways. For adults, the primary diagnostic question has to do with the nature of the individual's stuttering at the present time. That is, since stuttering begins in early childhood, for adults who come to our clinics the typical concern is not "Do I stutter?" but rather "Can I be helped?" As such, the diagnostic objectives are somewhat different than they would be for a child.

CHAPTER

3

Perspectives and Guidelines

I. APPROACHES TO THE TREATMENT OF STUTTERING

There is a wide array of published approaches available to the practicing professional for treating stuttering across the life span in both book and kit formats. We will not attempt to provide an inclusive list here. Two excellent sources for perusing available approaches include "Synopsis of Approaches to the Treatment of Stuttering" in Richard Culatta and Stanley A. Goldberg's (1995) book, *Stuttering Therapy: An Integrated Approach to Theory and Practice,* and "A Review of Therapies" in Meryl J. Wall and Florence L. Myers's (1995) book, *Clinical Management of Childhood Stuttering.* In addition, Ham's (1990) and Shapiro's (1999) textbooks both provide detailed explanations for teaching many of the techniques discussed in this chapter. Finally, in the most recent edition of his textbook, *Stuttering: An Integrated Approach to Its Nature and Treatment,* Barry Guitar (1998) provides a helpful description of the approaches used by a variety of well-known and influential clinicians. Within this discussion, Guitar includes a description of the two broad approaches to stuttering treatment which form the foundation for the various treatment programs developed by these specialists: the "speak more fluently" and "stutter more fluently" approaches, also known as "fluency shaping" and "stuttering modification," respectively. As we will discuss later, a number of clinicians, including ourselves, treat the problem of stuttering by using an integration of the two. We will briefly describe fluency shaping and stuttering modification approaches and then focus on the ways in which the key components of each approach can be combined to treat stuttering in a unified manner.

A. "Speak More Fluently" or Fluency Shaping Therapy

As the name implies, this fluency shaping (FS) approach focuses on increasing and maintaining fluent speech. The desired outcome of FS therapy is either spontaneous fluency (i.e., fluent speech produced without the conscious use of any strategies or controls learned in therapy) or controlled fluency (i.e., where the individual maintains fluency by utilizing therapy strategies to produce an altered speech pattern). Speech behavior is targeted, typically by building stutter-free speech within the clinic, beginning at simple phonologic/linguistic levels (e.g., sounds, syllables, or words) and building gradually toward conversational speech. Specific techniques or strategies are taught to show the client how to change overall speech patterns, with gradual reduction in the degree to which the alteration is exaggerated. The exact nature and names of these techniques may vary across clinic programs, but they yield the same end product: fluent speech characterized by a relatively reduced rate, continuous voicing, and minimal tension in the speech musculature.

Usually the strategies used to achieve this fluent or stutter-free speech are taught separately, but they also can be bundled under a broad term, such as "easy speech" for young clients. The techniques or strategies include rate reduction, which is primarily accomplished through prolonged or stretched vowels and phrasing (or chunking) and pausing; easy onset or slow, smooth initiation of speech; light or soft articulatory contact; and connecting sounds and syllables while moving forward in the flow of speech, usually through continuous voicing (keeping the voice "on" while talking).

In his instructional videotape and accompanying manual, *A Primer for Stuttering Therapy*, Schwartz (1999) offers excellent taped examples of FS or smooth speech strategies, and descriptions of ways to teach them to clients. At first, this stutter-free speech is produced in an exaggerated manner, and thus sounds extremely unnatural. Speech or fluency naturalness eventually becomes the main focus of therapy and is shaped to the extent that it sounds more natural to both the client and other significant listeners (e.g., through gradually increased rate and/or decreased prolongation). After fluency is achieved in the therapy environment, skills are transferred to extra-clinic environments (e.g., home and school). It is presumed that changes in emotional and attitudinal components will occur as fluency increases; thus, emotions and attitudes are not directly addressed. FS therapy tends to be highly structured, and improvement is quantified in the form of percentages of stuttered syllables or words at target phonologic/linguistic levels. Shapiro (1999) suggests, and we agree, that FS is an appropriate treatment approach when the person who stutters (1) does not avoid speaking or stuttering, (2) has positive attitudes and feelings about himself or herself as a communicator, and (3) responds positively to trial FS therapy.

B. "Stutter More Fluently" or Stuttering Modification Therapy

Stuttering modification (SM) therapy focuses more on improvements in overall communication than on fluent speech production. The goals of SM therapy are typically spontaneous fluency, controlled fluency, or unlike FS therapy, acceptable stuttering (i.e., perceivable stuttering that is less noticeable and severe and is acceptable to the person who stutters). In its strong form, SM therapy focuses on reducing fears and avoidances of speaking and/or stuttering, along with helping the client to gain an understanding of related feelings and attitudes and how to address them.

Over the years, SM therapy has come to include a strong emphasis on identification and modification of stuttered disruptions, along with the overall goal of reducing speech avoidance and fear. For clients to identify when and how they stutter and to utilize strategies for changing stuttered disruptions "on the fly" (i.e., as or before they produce them), an important goal in therapy is the development of behavioral awareness. In this context, behavioral awareness refers to a kinesthetic and proprioceptive sensitivity to the physical feelings associated with stuttering and using these feelings as a cue for changing the struggle and tension to either a smooth production or a stuttered disruption of relatively short duration and free of muscular tension and other associated behaviors (i.e., acceptable stuttering). Development of behavioral awareness requires a combination of motor and mental training, as described in more detail in later chapters.

C. Integrated Approaches

Integrated approaches include some combination of FS and SM procedures. The combination ranges from an emphasis on fluency shaping
with stuttering modification techniques implemented as needed to a
largely SM approach with some FS strategies added to assist clients in
achieving more spontaneous or controlled fluency. The combination
chosen must be a direct result of the outcome of the evaluation in which
the relative contributions of behavioral, emotional, and attitudinal components have been discerned for an individual who stutters. In general,
however, a client-centered integrated approach provides the individual
with a powerful toolbox of strategies for changing speech and improv-
ing communication. The goal for the client is to feel confident using the
variety of choices to maximize smooth, forward-moving speech. For
example, if using FS strategies does not consistently yield stutter-free
speech, then the client can continue to stutter, but can modify those instances of stuttering so as to make them acceptable to oneself. By providing clients with different but complementary techniques, concen-
trated perfect practice, and overall support, we hope to assist them in
developing the type of communication skill and style they desire.

II. ADDITIONAL GUIDELINES

Effective treatment is a product of comprehensive assessment of behavioral,
emotional, and attitudinal components of stuttering prior to and throughout
the therapeutic process. Examining and reexamining progress in all three
areas helps to maintain a clear focus on the client's needs and achievements
and sets the stage for continuous goal setting and evaluation. Involvement
of the client in every stage of therapy is critical. Therapy typically takes
longer and requires greater effort when a client is older or has been stuttering for a long time. The potential for formation of negative attitudes and
emotions and complex patterns of stuttering is greater and more resistant to
change. Hence, it is imperative that clients understand they are the most important member of the therapy team and be aware of and involved in setting
and modifying both short- and long-term goals and in evaluating progress.
The client is also instrumental in identifying who, when, and how others will
be involved in therapy, with the speech-language pathologist (SLP) acting
as the coach on the sidelines, giving information and guidelines and teaching skills as needed.

The process involved in creating a painting is a helpful analogy for the relationship between the SLP and client who stutters. The SLP provides the

frame, canvas, paints, brushes, cloths, and instructions that vary in depth and breadth as needed. The client provides the subject and ideas; selects the colors, shapes, and images; and paints the picture. Both the SLP and the client consider progress, discuss appropriate modifications and future steps, and cooperate to achieve the intended product. As the painting nears completion, the SLP becomes less and less involved in the process, remaining available to the client, but only as requested.

A. The Client Is the Focus

The focus on the client that occurs in individual therapy allows for maximum understanding of the client's stuttering and in-depth exploration of feelings, attitudes, and behaviors. Initially, individual therapy allows the SLP and client to develop rapport—a trusting, cooperative, and respectful relationship that facilitates disclosure and change. The establishment of a high level of rapport is necessary for therapy to progress (Schum, 1986). Once rapport is strongly established, it fluctuates around that high level as therapy continues. These fluctuations are a normal aspect of the therapeutic relationship and signify ups and downs in closeness, progress, independence, and motivation over the course of therapy. For example, when a client openly discloses feelings about stuttering such as sadness, fear, embarrassment, or even shame, rapport is at a high level. At these points in therapy, the client has entrusted the SLP with very personal feelings, increasing the client's vulnerability. After opening up, the client may then pull back somewhat, essentially waiting to see if his or her feelings will be respected and acknowledged by the SLP. Once the client is confident that his or her feelings are safe, rapport once again increases. As therapy draws to a conclusion, rapport begins to reduce, but it never reaches the level that preceded the first interaction between client and SLP. This decline is a sign of growing independence on the part of the client. Trust has not decreased, but the need for the SLP's input lessens as the painting nears completion. This sign indicates the client is ready to let go and function independently (Schum, 1986).

B. Setting the Agenda/Developing a Plan

Interactions with clients during the diagnostic process, particularly during the interview/discussion about their stuttering, provide the groundwork for setting the therapeutic agenda. SLPs often ask clients what they would like their speech to be like today, tomorrow, next week, next month, in six months, in a year, and so forth. SLPs talk about the different ways of talking (i.e., speech behaviors and techniques) that clients could try, they model them, ask clients to try them out, and obtain their reactions. It is important to draw from each client's interests and skills to help him or her understand what it takes to change speech.

We often compare learning to talk—and learning to talk in a new way—to playing a musical instrument or a sport, building a collection, constructing a puzzle or model, painting a picture, or mastering a subject in school. We also discuss how the way we talk is influenced by how we feel and what we think. We may begin this conversation by discussing good and bad days and what affects them—our health, amount of sleep, schedules, interactions with others, performance at work, in school, sports, and so forth. We then apply this to our discussion of talking.

Some clients may not respond initially or indepth to the types of open-ended inquiries suggested above. For these clients, and for added insight into clients who do respond more fully, specific types of behaviors, feelings, and attitudes may be presented and evaluated. For example, use of the Modified Erickson Scale of Communication Attitude (24) (CAI, commonly refered to as the Communication Attitude Index) CAI for adults and the CAT-R for children allows the client to give a true/false response to statements about talking. Examining checklists that contain various types of situations in which clients typically talk is also helpful (e.g., Cooper & Cooper, 1985). If, in addition to a true/false type of response, the client provides a numerical or verbal rating of the situation (e.g., 0 = no problem to 5 = very difficult speaking situation, "not important" to "extremely important"), additional insight may be gained without the client needing to talk a great deal. When working with children, it is helpful to have them peruse magazines, looking for pictures and other representations of situations in which they communicate. Selected items are sorted according to the context (e.g., home, school, little league, scouts) and then according to difficulty. Items are arranged on pages of a notebook and descriptors added based on the client's input. Having pictorial cues often stimulates further discussion and disclosure by the child.

Regardless of age, the client, from the onset of therapy, should have a notebook in which to collect materials, chart progress, write or depict (for nonreaders) homework assignments, provide results and feedback, and log ideas, feelings, and thoughts. For children, keep a supply of notebooks of varying sizes, shapes, colors, and types, allowing the client to choose from among them. All of the notebooks contain pockets for loose materials that have not yet been added to the permanent pages and lots of blank paper. Children especially like to title their notebook and illustrate or decorate it as they see fit. We encourage them to keep their notebooks in their backpacks for easy access during the day and evening. Some clients have a larger and a smaller notebook, using the larger one for permanent entries and ideas, thoughts, and feelings they wish to share with others (e.g., SLP, parents, teachers). The smaller notebook is often a more private collection of materials and personal entries that are "under construction" and not ready to be shared with others. The authors have found this to be helpful in reinforcing the concept of the client as his or her own clinician and expert about stuttering, giving the client control and leadership when it comes to the therapeutic process.

C. Prioritizing

It has been our experience that one of the contributing factors to failure in fluency treatment is a lack of emphasis placed on the importance and pervasiveness of communication in the lives of all people, including, of course, school-age clients who stutter. Fluency therapy is often seen as one small part of the client's incredibly full and busy life, rather than as an integral part of nearly every activity in which he or she participates. It should be apparent, from the therapeutic procedures included thus far, that we take the time to familiarize ourselves with every facet of our client's daily experiences and the role of communication in those experiences. By addressing the client's behavioral, emotional, and attitudinal concerns holistically, both the importance of communication and the practical utility of fluency therapy are demonstrated. We strive to equip the client with tools that enhance communication while also promoting self-awareness, independence, and even organizational skills. The tasks involved in fluency therapy require careful self-examination; detailed analyses of daily routines and interactions; and careful planning, execution, monitoring, and modifying of therapeutic goals. Improved communication skills help to bolster confidence and encourage exploration of new experiences. If we help clients to understand and appreciate the gains they have made in communicating and the applicability of such gains to other facets of their daily lives, they will appreciate and apply skills learned far beyond the brief time spent directly in therapy.

In taking such a holistic approach, knowing and understanding priorities is critical. One reason why so many of us avoid looking at the big picture in any given situation is that it appears overwhelming and impossible to control. Deciding where to start may appear elusive. We approach this problem by, once again, returning to the results of our ongoing assessment of the behavioral, emotional, and attitudinal components of stuttering. We listen carefully to the outcome of our discussions with the client concerning short-term and long-term goals. The results of trial therapy during which various techniques are demonstrated and attempted by the client are also useful. From these sources, we generate objectives and rationale, and we select specific procedures for therapy with our clients. Following are several rules of thumb to keep in mind.

1. **Start Where the Client Is.** Even if we might prioritize the client's needs and likely objectives differently, by working on a goal deemed critical to the client, we generate hope, success, and the level of rapport between client and SLP necessary for both short- and long-term success.

2. **Be Practical.** Remember that clients will be much more motivated if they see the application of what they are learning beyond the particular context in which the skill is taught. Discuss how the technique can be used in many different settings. Talk about the short- and long-term applications of the skill from the beginning. Have the client immediately try the skill outside of therapy, carefully planning the context and steps that will be taken for the assignment. The client must be completely involved in the planning process so that he or she feels and takes ownership of the skill and the responsibility for practicing it.

3. **Constantly Reevaluate the Plan.** Reevaluation does not mean constant changes in the plan. Rather, by continuously examining for whom, what, when, where, and why the long- and short-term goals are established, you maintain focus on the client, the therapeutic plan, and progress across areas. After each session, take a look at all goals and document results and observations.

4. **Remember to Put the Client First.** Avoid the natural tendency, as the expert, to do, make, or decide for the client. Where is the client in the therapy process? What is the client ready for? What is important to the client? At times, it feels as though progress is slower when we follow our client's lead, rather than insisting that he or she follow ours. If we run ahead, rattling off a list of instructions and insisting that the client hurry and catch up, we have, in essence, intercepted the ball and run with it, leaving the client on the other side of the playing field, empty handed. By focusing on the fact that

we serve our clients and that our ultimate goal is their independence, we will remember to put our clients first.

D. Rapport and Motivation

Earlier, we addressed variations in rapport that occur naturally over the course of therapy. Fluctuations in therapeutic intensity are the cause of such variations in rapport. Initially, when rapport is high, the client is motivated to address and make changes in fluency. If we have done a good job putting the client in the driver's seat, then motivation is enhanced and the client is committed and enthusiastic. Over time, as with any change that requires commitment, practice, and perseverance, therapeutic intensity will fluctuate. It is important that we observe and respect such fluctuations, being careful to maximize intense periods and accept more modest efforts and gains during less intense periods.

An analogy to exercise may be helpful here. It has been demonstrated that alterations between more and less intense exercise bouts are beneficial to cardiovascular fitness, muscle toning, and weight reduction. Less intense bouts help to reenergize us for bouts of greater exercise intensity. They also give us (and our muscles) a break from more taxing efforts. In fluency therapy, variations in intensity have a similar effect. Less intense periods can be rewarding, reenergizing, and used to take a breath, evaluate progress, and prepare for a more intense period of concentration on therapeutic goals. They also help the client to prepare for dismissal from therapy, yielding opportunities to evaluate how well changes are maintained during breaks or less intense efforts.

Most SLPs have had experiences with clients who, no matter how hard they try, are less motivated in therapy. For children, this may occur at the beginning of therapy if parents and/or teachers are more interested in the client changing his or her speech than the client is. For adults, lack of motivation may be an indication that a significant other in the client's life (e.g., a spouse or employer) is the main force behind the client's initial contact with the clinic, as well as attendance at subsequent sessions. With this scenario, we focus on the clients' perceptions and spend time gaining an appreciation of their points of view, discussing more general issues and goals and establishing critical rapport. As a result, we are often able to help the client over this initial reluctance.

Reduced motivation is even more likely to occur later in therapy when the novelty wears off and gains are either less pronounced or take more work to accomplish. This is evident in some clients who become like weekend athletes, who only play a sport on the weekend (i.e., during therapy sessions), committing little time or energy to it during the week (i.e., outside of therapy). This is first exemplified by incomplete homework with frequent excuses that range from "I forgot," to "I don't know how," to "I didn't have enough time." When this occurs, we first evaluate, along with our clients, whether the short-term goals being addressed are appropriate, including the particular tasks and outcomes selected. We then address motivation in therapy directly, analogizing it to other commitments and tasks in the client's life (e.g., schoolwork, sports, hobbies). It is helpful to acknowledge that we do not expect that the client will always be motivated or always complete agreed-upon assignments. We may use examples from our own experiences to show our understanding and empathy for the client's current feelings.

Following these discussions we make decisions, along with our clients and other members of the therapy team as appropriate, about the next step. At times a client simply needs to talk about motivation and its natural fluctuations and to be reenergized in therapy (in essence, given a pep talk). It may be decided that particular goals need a rest while we focus on others. At other times, a break from therapy is needed. In each of these situations, we draw up a contract with the client, specifying what has been accomplished, what remains, short-term modifications, and long-term goals. At times, the intensity of therapy may be decreased. For example, a break from focusing on speech behaviors may be instituted with the client continuing to log thoughts, feelings, and experiences over a one-month period. In some cases, it may be decided that a complete break from therapy should be taken for two or three months. An appointment is scheduled to occur at the conclusion of the break. At that time, the client, SLP, and others as needed will meet and decide upon the next step. During the break, the client is free to contact the SLP to reinitiate therapy or simply to keep in touch. Whenever a contract is created, the terms should be clearly specified and a written version signed by all those involved.

There are times when a client appears to need a reduction in therapeutic intensity or a temporary break from therapy, and others (e.g., parents) are not in favor of such changes. In these cases, it is important that we counsel significant others, giving them the rationale for the changes, explaining the purpose and terms of the contract, and assuring them that the break is temporary and will be reevaluated on a particular date. We also talk about our previous experiences with contracts for modifying or taking breaks in therapy and about the positive consequences we are seeking. Oftentimes, a short-term change will pay off in the long term in the areas of self-responsibility, motivation, and overall progress. For some clients, this may be a "two steps forward, one step back" type of experience. For others, it may be more like a vacation or refueling stop that helps them to gather energy and motivation for the road ahead. If we view it positively, stay in touch, and follow up, this can be a useful tool in therapeutic progress.

III. CONCLUSION

Once treatment for stuttering is determined to be warranted and recommended, the clinician needs to consider a number of important factors. For example, what are the available treatment approaches? How do they differ and how are they similar? What approach or combination of approaches is the best for this particular client? What rationale will I provide to the client (or the client's parents) for the approach I will use? In addition, general issues of treatment plan development, such as appropriate goal selection and prioritization, the importance of remaining client focused, establishing rapport, and promoting client motivation are significant components of stuttering intervention.

CHAPTER

4

Therapy for the Preschool Child

In Chapter 2, we outlined procedures for assessing and diagnosing stuttering across the lifespan. In general, we specified the behaviors (speech and associated), emotions/feelings, and thoughts/attitudes that are critical at various junctures in normal development and in the epigenesis of stuttering. For preschoolers, the nature of the speech disfluency and the child's reactions to it; the likelihood for recovery; and the concerns, reactions, and interaction styles of caregivers were highlighted. Methods for assessment of the child's developmental status, including speech, language, hearing, and cognitive abilities, as well as temperament and social skills, were considered. A comprehensive evaluation allows the clinician to gain an understanding of the child's current fluency and developmental status in relation to his or her environment. The resulting information may then be utilized to make critical decisions for planning and implementing therapy. The first decision needs to be whether therapy is indicated and recommended.

I. THERAPY DECISIONS BASED ON EVALUATION RESULTS

A. Is Therapy Indicated?

1. No Therapy Is Indicated. Therapy is typically not indicated when the evaluation reveals that the child's speech and related behaviors are not consistent with a diagnosis of stuttering. Frequently, parents are concerned about occasional repetitions of sounds, syllables, and/or monosyllabic whole words, particularly when the child is excited, tired, and/or upset. Parents of these children typically tell us that they "thought it was normal" but "just wanted to make sure." In response, we provide them with information about general development and disfluency in young children and remain available for future consultation should their child's speech fluency change. Case Example 4-1 serves to illustrate this point.

Case Example 4-1

We were recently contacted by an occupational therapist who was concerned about her son, Mark (their first child), who began to stutter (i.e., use repeated syllables and monosyllabic whole words) one week previously. She informed us that she was not sure whether she should be concerned and that her husband felt that Mark would soon outgrow it. We gave the parents the option of coming to the clinic for an evaluation so that we could discuss their observations, Mark's potential risk for continued stuttering, and strategies for responding to the stuttering at home. The parents decided to bring Mark for an evaluation that was scheduled to occur three weeks later.

During the evaluation, we observed that Mark's symptoms were consistent with children who do not stutter and that he had none of the potential risk factors (see Chapter 2) for chronic stuttering. We provided this information to his parents, answered their questions, and left the door open for further evaluations if they noticed behaviors more typical of stuttering. They expressed relief and were thankful for the information we provided about typical speech, language, and fluency abilities in children of Mark's age.

---

2. Therapy May Be Indicated. The situation in Case Example 4-1 frequently occurs when a child is stuttering on occasion and, when present, the stuttering is more frequent and severe than is typical of the speech of children who do not stutter. In addition, the stuttering has typically persisted for less than 14 months and is sporadic (e.g., Ambrose & Yairi, 1999; Throneburg & Yairi, 2001). In other words, these children show fewer, rather than more, of the risk factors identified in Chapter 2. Their parents tend to be at least mildly concerned and want to prevent, if at all possible, the stuttering from worsening. In these types of cases, we believe that the best approach is a combination of indirect therapy, in which parents are taught to provide fluency-facilitating models for their children, and periodic reevaluations (about every 3 months) of the child's stuttering. In subsequent portions of this chapter, we will describe indirect therapy procedures in more detail. Periodic reevaluations help us to "keep tabs" on the child so that we may be available if the stuttering worsens, document changes over time, answer the parents' questions, and help them to respond positively to the child's stuttering if it continues.

One useful procedure that we use to follow children's stuttering between evaluations is to have parents complete the daily stuttering tracking form, as shown in Appendix A. Each parent is given a copy of the form and asked to rate, on a daily basis, the average severity of the child's stuttering. Space is provided for comments and questions and other information parents wish to share. We recommend that parents make their ratings at the end of the day, after they put their child to bed and/or just before they retire for the night. Parents have informed us that they find the procedure easy and quick (1 to 2 minutes per day) and that it allows them to reflect upon, and have a better understanding of, their child's stuttering. The use of this procedure is an example of a counseling technique called binding, in which clients are given "activities in order to focus their nervous energy into something constructive" (Schum, 1986, p. 44). For parents of children who stutter, the activity gives them something to do to help their child at a time when the outcome of the child's stuttering is unknown and most suggestions to parents are things "not to do" rather than things "to do."

By keeping tabs on children who stutter with periodic reevaluations and by being available to parents as needed, we are also ready to implement more structured indirect and/or direct methods for treating the stuttering if they become warranted or the parents desire to begin therapy immediately. These methods will be discussed in greater detail later. Note that the majority of children we see between the ages of 2 and 4 years fit into this "maybe" category. Stuttering is present, along with several other risk factors, but the weight of the evidence suggests transient stuttering. Case Example 4-2 provides a rather typical scenario.

Case Example 4-2

Susan, a 3-year-old, had been stuttering on and off for 6 months. She sometimes repeats the first sound/syllable of a sentence up to 10 times when telling a story or when she is excited about a recent event. Her grandmother said that Susan's father had done something very similar when he was a preschooler, but it "went away before he started kindergarten."

The evaluation revealed that Susan's language skills were well above age-level expectations. She tended to repeat the first sound/syllable of sentences when she was excited, interrupted others, and/or was talking about events removed in time and/or context. We noticed that Susan continued to talk unabashedly except when her parents interrupted or asked her to slow down. At those times, she lowered her eyes and briefly stopped talking. Her parents expressed frustration with the long strings of repetitions, and sometimes they finished Susan's words or instructed her to slow down. They reported that Susan's stuttering was inconsistent, disappearing for days at a time and then reappearing "out of the blue."

We provided the parents with information and handouts about developmental stuttering from the Stuttering Foundation of America (SFA) (see Appendix C) and asked them to (a) refrain from interrupting or telling Susan to slow down; (b) model relaxed communication by inserting longer pauses between utterances in their own speech; and (c) reinforce the content of Susan's utterances. We demonstrated these techniques and encouraged her parents to do the same. Following the evaluation, the parents continued to track Susan's stuttering and returned to the clinic every 3 months for a full year. During this time, the frequency and duration of Susan's repetitions decreased, and the length of fluent speech periods (i.e., days, then weeks, then months) increased. At her last two evaluations, Susan's speech fluency was similar to that of normally fluent children both in the clinic and at home.

---

3. Therapy Is Indicated. When children are clearly stuttering, their parents are concerned, and the weight of the evidence suggests that they are at risk for continuing to stutter. As outlined earlier, we enroll these children in therapy as soon as possible (see Case Example 4-3).

Case Example 4-3

Frank, a 4-year-old, had been stuttering for over 2 years when his parents brought him to the clinic for an evaluation. He had been identified during a screening of speech, language, and hearing at his preschool. Stuttering was noticed in both conversation and single-word productions. Frank prolonged the first sound of many words, increasing his pitch, blinking his eyes, and covering his mouth as he did so. His parents reported that this behavior had been present, off and on, from age 2 or 3, but it occurred almost all of the time for the past year. They had expressed concern to their pediatrician who told them not to worry unless it persisted in kindergarten. Frank's maternal uncle reportedly stutters as an adult but less severely than he did in elementary school.

Results of Frank's evaluation revealed age-appropriate speech and language abilities and concern on the part of both Frank ("I don't talk like other kids") and his parents ("We feel so badly when he struggles like that"). We immediately enrolled Frank in therapy using a combination of direct therapy with him and indirect strategies with his parents (to be described later in this chapter).

B. If Therapy Is Indicated, What Approach Should Be Taken?

If children demonstrate an awareness of their stuttering, and particularly if their reactions to the stuttering are negative, we will most likely take a direct approach to therapy in which speech and stuttering (usually called "bumpy" or "sticky" speech) are directly discussed and modified. Parents are given indirect strategies to implement in the clinic and at home. If awareness is minimal or absent, but risk factors strongly suggest possible continuation of stuttering, we often start by initiating indirect therapy in which clinicians implement, and train parents to implement, techniques that help to facilitate fluency in young children. Activities build from easier to more difficult levels of linguistic and pragmatic complexity as children's fluency increases. We will discuss these techniques in greater detail shortly.

II. DEVELOPING THE TREATMENT PLAN

A. Considering Behavioral, Emotional, and Attitudinal Components

As outlined in Chapter 2 and suggested in the preceding portion of this chapter, all behavioral, emotional, and attitudinal components of stuttering are considered in the development of a treatment plan. With preschoolers who stutter, the behavioral components tend to be the main consideration. These include stutteringlike disfluencies and their attributes, including frequency, type, duration, and number of iterations, as well as any nonspeech behaviors (e.g., eye blinking and head movement). Many preschoolers evince these symptoms without any apparent emotional and/or attitudinal reactions. When this is the case, therapy focuses on providing children with speaking environments that encourage and make fluent speech production more likely (e.g., slow-paced and noninterruptive environments with predictable conversational interactions). We call this indirect fluency therapy. It may be conducted one on one with children and their families or in groups of parents and children.

Some children show emotional reactions that consist mainly of surprise or fleeting frustration at their inability to talk, in addition to the speech and nonspeech behaviors just described (Guitar, 1998). Attitudinal reactions, if any, tend to be restricted to the perception that speaking is "hard for me," similar to a young child's perception that coloring, riding a bike, or any other skill may be difficult to accomplish (e.g., Williams, 1982). We find that children who are frustrated and/or perceive speaking as difficult are often those who have had tremendous success with speaking (e.g., early, prolific talkers, especially girls) prior to the onset of stuttering, and/or have sensitive temperaments characterized by higher levels of awareness of, and less tolerance for, "mistakes" or difficulties while talking (or doing anything else, for that matter). When there is evidence of negative emotional and/or attitudinal responses to stuttering by children, we often combine indirect therapy focused on facilitating fluency with exercises, implemented by clinicians and parents, that help children to be more tolerant of making mistakes in general, and while speaking in particular. Case Example 4-4 focuses on a young child who fits this profile.

Case Example 4-4

At age $2\frac{1}{2}$ years, Shelby was a frequent and proficient talker. According to her parents, one day "out of the blue," Shelby started to block completely every time she spoke. They could think of nothing that might have triggered it. They were concerned that Shelby sometimes refused to talk, talked in a whisper, or cried when she struggled. On several occasions, Shelby asked her mother, "Mommy, why can't I talk?"

During the evaluation, Shelby demonstrated all of the behaviors her parents described and, at one point, burst into tears, climbed under a table, and refused to come out saying, "No more talking." Her parents reported that Shelby "is very particular about everything" (her clothes, hair, toys, meals, etc.) and "becomes easily frustrated whenever she can't do anything the first time" (e.g., dress herself, color, complete a puzzle). Her parents said they "don't know why she's like this," and they reported that their efforts to joke with her or ease her frustration were unsuccessful.

Shelby's evaluation revealed an absence of risk factors for chronic stuttering with the exception of the stuttering behavior itself and her negative reactions to it. Her parents were observed to listen carefully—never interrupting and complimenting the content of her utterances.

We enrolled Shelby in weekly therapy. The initial focus was to help Shelby tolerate her own mistakes. We modeled "mistakes" while building with blocks, completing puzzles, coloring, dressing dolls, making cookies, and so forth, and we used self-talk to comment upon and respond to our own mistakes with acceptance (e.g., "That's okay. I'll try again. Everyone makes mistakes sometimes. You have to keep trying. Mistakes are a good way to learn."). Shelby was distressed when we were upset and quickly began to use our comments to reassure us and then, within a month, to comment upon her own "mistakes." Shelby's parents used similar self-talk outside of the clinic. Shelby's stuttering subsided completely by the end of the month and was absent at all follow-up evaluations.

B. Working with Children Who Are Likely to Recover

Recall that children who are likely to recover from stuttering are those who are younger, are fewer months poststuttering onset, have no family history of persistent stuttering, produce fewer SLDs which fluctuate over time, and evince few if any reactions to stuttering. Gender is also a consideration. More females (85%) recover than males (69%) (Ambrose & Yairi, 1999; Throneburg & Yairi, 2001). Children who are likely to recover are those for whom therapy may be necessary and to whom we provide therapy with the objective of helping the child and family through a period during which the child's stuttering is excessive, and the possibility exists (however remote) that stuttering may continue. Our goals are to maximize communication efforts and ease, while minimizing fluency disruptors. This may be accomplished through several therapy options, including indirect, direct, or a combination of the two approaches.

1. **Therapy Options.** When the weight of evidence suggests that a child will recover, the next decision we make is whether to employ indirect or direct treatment with the child and family. Sometimes, a combination of the two, or a progression from indirect to direct methods, is indicated as therapy proceeds.

   a. Indirect therapy. This type is typically implemented first for children who are likely to recover from stuttering. By indirect, we mean that children's stuttering, as well as their general speaking abilities, are not directly addressed. In other words, we will not be teaching children to talk differently or to recognize and change their stuttering and related behavior. The focus is on adjusting the contexts in which communication occurs to facilitate easy, effortless, and fluent speech. Parents, as trained by clinicians, are the most important agents of change. They are the primary role models and "experts" about their children and what is best for them.

   The first step in indirect therapy involves assessment of parental models during interaction with their children. The purpose of this assessment is to determine a starting place for implementing such therapy. Behaviors such as turn-taking (e.g., pausing, interrupting, eye contact, body posture, balance of turns), rate of speech, complexity of child-directed speech and language, frequency and level of questioning, and the warmth or supportiveness of communicative interaction are analyzed.

Parents are asked to identify situations and/or behaviors (by the child and others) that seem to elicit more stuttering by their child. In a similar manner, the child's own speaking patterns are analyzed to focus on the stuttering, as well as characteristics of the child's conversational output (e.g., frequency and complexity of speech and language, concomitant concerns) and turn-taking abilities. Results of the assessment of parent-child interactions are then used to identify those behaviors to target in indirect therapy (e.g., frequent interruptions by the child and/or parents, one speaker dominating conversation, rapid parental speech rate, frequent questions by parents and/or child, inattention to the child when he speaks). One example of the application of this method is presented in a study by Guitar et al. (1992) in which parental rate, interruptions, amount of talking, and frequency of positive and negative utterances were targeted. Parents of a 5-year-old who was stuttering were trained to modify these behaviors over the course of 5 months of treatment. The results included decreases in speech rates by both parents and decreases in stuttering by their daughter.

Indirect therapy typically involves sporadic sessions in the clinic. The clinician may see the family for the initial evaluation, one or more training sessions for indirect techniques, and periodic follow-up evaluations (e.g., monthly, then bimonthly, then semiannually). When we have two to five children of similar age and stuttering histories, we often form parent-child fluency therapy groups. Parents meet separately from children for support, information exchange, modeling, and training of fluency-facilitating skills by the SLP. They also watch the children's group and practice their techniques with their own child and with all the children and parents. In the children's group, the SLP utilizes fluency-facilitating strategies in activities that gradually increase in linguistic, contextual, and conversational (e.g., turn-taking) demands for the children. They also serve as models for the parents to observe and emulate when they join the children.

b. Direct therapy. This type involves a number of different levels of attention to the child's speech and/or stuttering. At the simplest level, which is typically initiated when indirect therapy is producing few changes, children are taught to recognize and then produce slow (e.g., "turtle") and recognize fast (e.g., "rabbit") speech. Rabbit speech is characterized as too fast—making it hard to talk and/or be understood. In contrast, turtle speech is portrayed as easy to understand and produce. At a more complex (second) level, children are taught to contrast "sticky" or "bumpy" speech with "smooth" or "easy" speech. Turtle speech is still the focus, but children now evaluate how smooth or easy, versus bumpy or sticky, their productions are. If further attention is needed, instructions for production of "stretched" speech (i.e., slightly prolonged) and/or "soft touches" (i.e., light articulatory contacts) are used to help the children "keep speech moving." This third level includes more attention to how we produce our sounds, words, and sentences.

Direct therapy is combined with indirect therapy to maximize benefits within and, more importantly, outside of the clinic. Parents are instructed to implement indirect therapy techniques with their children at all levels and stages of therapy. When indicated, parents may also be instructed to model the use of direct therapy techniques and practice them with their children, particularly when additional experience outside of therapy is needed for carryover of easy and/or smooth speech. We do not, however, teach parents to praise or punish their children's speech verbally according to the quality of *fluency* produced, as is central to some current therapy approaches. We believe it is important that parents not be put in a position of evaluating their child's fluency as correct or incorrect. This may result in communication becoming an unpleasant experience for young children who quickly learn that there are good and bad ways of talking, and that their parents do not want to hear them speak when they stutter. We prefer that parents focus more on the content of their child's production (i.e., what he or she says) than on speech fluency and provide models of talking that reduce communicative demands and encourage their child to talk, whether they stutter or not. Other persons in the child's environment, such as grandparents, teachers, and daycare personnel, may also be involved in indirect or direct therapy as warranted by the child's needs and level of treatment.

2. Treatment Objectives.

   a. Role of Clinician. The clinician's role in therapy is to provide parents with information, model appropriate interaction styles and techniques, and assist parents with monitoring of the child's stuttering, and their own use of fluency-facilitating strategies outside of the therapy setting. Once treatment becomes direct, the clinician instructs the child in the target techniques, ensures that parents understand the rationale for therapeutic approaches and activities, monitors parents' abilities to implement indirect procedures within the clinic and at home, and assigns and monitors homework activities (indirect and/or direct) to be completed by parents and/or children. An example of a typical homework assignment near the beginning of indirect therapy is presented in Case Example 4-5.

Case Example 4-5

During the 2-week period between Joey's evaluation and the start of therapy, his parents tracked his stuttering, took notes, and commented on speaking situations (see Appendix B for the appropriate form) and family activities. At his first therapy session, the SLP gathered additional information about Joey's fluency and about the situations the parents had noted. The parents observed the SLP interacting with Joey using a slow rate and careful turn-taking (i.e., pausing and avoiding the chance to interrupt) while they played. They then practiced using similar models in interaction with Joey and the SLP during a variety of activities.

Afterwards, the parents noted that the changes were easier to make in structured than in more open-ended activities. The SLP then helped the parents to identify a few simple, structured homework activities during which they would make changes (i.e., practice slowing their rates and taking turns). Joey's parents selected daily rides in the car to and from preschool during which they played guessing games (e.g., "I see something red. Is it a _____?") to start practicing their indirect skills with Joey. By focusing on a homework situation that was already a part of the family routine, the parents were able to modify their interactions to facilitate Joey's fluency without adding another event to their already busy schedules. The frequency and complexity of homework scenarios were then expanded as therapy progressed.

---

b. Role of Parents. The roles of parents include commitment to the therapeutic process and implementation of indirect and/or direct techniques in the home as prescribed by the clinician. Parents provide information about the child's stuttering, his or her response to (in)direct fluency-facilitating strategies, and the outcome of various homework assignments as illustrated in Case Example 4-5. Parents are advised that they are more important to the therapeutic process than the SLP, because they spend much more time with their child and know their child much better than the SLP. In addition, the success of indirect therapy depends upon the parents, because it is largely implemented outside of the clinic setting.

The daily stuttering tracking form (see Appendix A), described earlier, is one means we employ to enlist parents in the monitoring of their child's stuttering and related behavior. In addition, we provide each family with a journal in which the tracking sheets are inserted, along with notes from therapy, instructions for activities, and pages for parent notes as well as notes from others (e.g., teachers, babysitters, grandparents). Examples of journal entries for two preschoolers, one in indirect and one in direct therapy, are provided in Case Examples 4-6 and 4-7.

c. Role of Others. The roles of others depend upon the family constellation and the schedules of individual children. Most of the time, parents are responsible for telling others what they have learned about their child's stuttering, what they are doing to help, and what others may do. Literature and videotapes from the SFA, specifically designed for parents and/or teachers, are indispensable in these efforts. Appendix C contains a list of materials and contact information for the SFA and other useful sources.

In some families, older siblings (e.g., teenagers) or grandparents (see Case Example 4-7) may assist in caring for the child on a daily basis. When this is the case, they also may be asked to monitor the child's stuttering (e.g., with the tracking forms) and implement indirect fluency-facilitating strategies. Teachers or daycare personnel may also be involved, with input ranging from daily conversations with caregivers who transport the children, to the provision of written journal entries. When chil-

---

Case Example 4-6

Three-year-old Jenny is receiving indirect fluency therapy in the clinic with the SLP using a slowed rate and structured turn-taking at gradually increasing levels of linguistic demand. Jenny's parents are implementing the same fluency-facilitating strategies at home, and her preschool teacher is monitoring Jenny's fluency. The following are entries during one week of therapy.

SLP: Jenny is fluent during structured turn-taking activities (e.g., "Go Fish," "Simon Says," and "Don't Break the Ice") and when required to respond with single words, phrases, or short, descriptive sentences. She has difficulty taking turns and speaking fluently during unstructured conversation and/or free play. We will work on conversation during structured play (e.g., with the doll house, kitchen set, and veterinary kit) next week.

Mother: I am able to keep my rate slow and do not interrupt Jenny when we are setting the table, emptying the dishwasher, and making cookies at home. I don't notice any stuttering at those times. When my husband reads to Jenny at night, he practices talking more slowly. Jenny mostly listens and doesn't say much when he reads, but she is very calm and relaxed. She seems to love the one-on-one time each of us is spending with her.

Preschool teacher: I don't notice any stuttering when we are having story or circle time. During show and tell, Jenny is fluent as long as the other children are looking at and listening to her. She becomes frustrated and starts to stutter when interrupted. I try to encourage all the children to wait their turns and look and listen when others are talking.

---

dren who stutter are being seen by more than one SLP (e.g., across school and private settings) or when other communication concerns are being addressed, services are coordinated so that each SLP provides information about objectives, activities, accomplishments, and recommendations. This information is

---

Case Example 4-7

Peter, who is 4 years old, has been working on producing turtle speech in structured activities with his SLP. They take turns using their turtle speech while describing objects pulled from a grab bag, assembling Legos™, and arranging pictures in sequence. The SLP reinforces Peter for using turtle speech and asks him to "try again" when he uses rabbit speech. His father, grandmother (who cares for him while his father is at work), and his SLP provided the following entries in his journal.

SLP: Peter consistently knows the difference between turtle and rabbit speech in his own and in my speech during structured activities and when I produce them in conversation. He is able to produce turtle speech consistently during structured activities such as playing "grab bag," putting Lego™ cars and trucks together, and playing "Turtle Says." If he forgets, he is able to modify his productions. He produces very few disfluencies during these activities. During free play, he quickly notes my rabbit speech, but often misses his own. When I "catch him," he smiles and tries again, using his turtle speech successfully.

Father: Peter seems to be able to use his turtle speech when he wants to. I don't think he likes to be reminded of it, so I try not to say anything. He likes to catch me using rabbit speech. When he does, I ask him to show me how to do it, and he does a good job. He says I need a lot of help!

Grandmother: Whenever Peter and I are alone together, I never notice any stuttering. He talks pretty slowly and is relaxed. He knows I understand. Peter stutters a lot more when he is playing with other children, especially when they are all excited or fighting over a toy. He talks a lot faster then.

---

often added to the child's journal, which travels in his or her backpack and is monitored by parents who are responsible for making sure the journal is transported to all necessary participants in the child's total treatment plan. The journal entries for Case Example 4-8 are from a child who receives SLP services at preschool and periodic reevaluations in our clinic.

Case Example 4-8

Michael was initially evaluated by a SLP who began indirect fluency therapy with him at his preschool. He continued to exhibit tension and pitch elevations during prolongations, so she began direct therapy after a few weeks. She contacted us for additional ideas and suggestions and for periodic evaluations to make sure she was on the right track. The SLP, Michael's mother, and his preschool teacher each provide journal entries and complete tracking forms. Here are a few examples.

Mother: Michael's stuttering has improved this week. I think the problems he had earlier were tied to the beginning of the school year. He was nervous about his new teacher, the new kids in his class, and going to speech therapy. I think he was afraid to leave the classroom. Now, he just loves school and speech therapy and seems to be happier. He stutters at a 2 or 3 severity at home most of the time. When he does stutter, though, he still pushes the sound out really hard. Sometimes I tell him to relax, even though I probably shouldn't.

Preschool teacher: I have also noticed a decrease in Michael's stuttering. I have tried to talk slowly and encourage all the children to take turns. I think the whole classroom is a bit more manageable lately! Michael has decreased from a 4 or 5 on the severity scale to a 2 or 3 in recent weeks. One child imitated him when he had a long stutter the other day, and I talked to that child privately. I don't want Michael or any other child in my class teased.

SLP: Michael is stuttering less and is less apprehensive about coming to see me. He didn't like turtle speech very much, but he really likes to use stretchy speech with the assistance of an elasticized cloth band. He does best at the single-word or carrier phrase levels. I have been modeling "stretches" in my spontaneous speech and he enjoys "catching" me "stretching," because I let him earn stickers for being a "good listener." He occasionally uses a stretch in spontaneous conversation, and I reinforce it. Next week when you come in, Mrs. R., I would like Michael to teach you how he stretches his speech, so that he can start practicing with you at home.

C. Working with Children Who Are Likely to Persist

1. **Therapy Options.** Indirect, direct, or a combination of the two approaches to therapy are applied when the results of our assessment suggest that a child is at risk for continued stuttering. The main differences between the approaches we take with these children, as compared with those who are likely to recover, are the frequency of therapy, how rapidly we progress from indirect to direct therapy, and the intensity of services (both within and outside of the clinic). There is not a set formula for making these decisions. Rather, by observing closely, obtaining quantitative and qualitative data, and working closely with the family, we tailor therapy to the individual child's needs.

   a. Indirect therapy. This type of therapy is implemented when the child is stuttering and at risk for continuing (with many chronicity risk factors) but shows little awareness of, or concern about, stuttering. Thus, our first level of treatment is to determine what aspects of daily life and conversational interaction may be challenging the child's speech fluency as discussed previously. We then address these challenges with the assistance of parents and significant others in the child's environment. We may see the family weekly for one to two months during this early stage of therapy. If, in a month or two, indirect treatment is ineffective (i.e., either the stuttering worsens or shows no change), we will move to direct therapy, while continuing indirect strategies outside of the clinic.

   b. Direct treatment. This type of therapy begins with the simplest level at which children are taught to contrast and produce rabbit and turtle speech, with a focus on increased use of "turtle talk" and decreased use or elimination of rabbit speech. We will typically stay at this level for 4 to 6 weeks before making a decision regarding progression to the next level at which children learn about sticky or bumpy, versus smooth or easy speech, and are taught to repeat their words, phrases, and sentences that contained sticky or bumpy speech using turtle speech. Once again, we implement this stage for 4 to 6 weeks, monitoring progress. If the child worsens or does not improve, we move to the third level of direct therapy where our attention focuses on how fluent and stuttered speech is produced and techniques for preventing or modifying stuttering when it occurs (e.g., prolonged or stretched speech). We are most likely to progress to this level when children continue to exhibit tension during production of SLDs or are frustrated with their inability to communicate. Direct techniques continue to be accompanied by indirect methods implemented by clinicians, parents, and others.

2. Treatment Objectives.

a. Role of Clinician. The clinician's role with children who are at risk for continued stuttering is identical to that described for children who are likely to recover. Briefly, for indirect treatment, clinicians provide parents with information, model techniques, and assist them with implementation and monitoring outside of the therapy setting. Once treatment becomes direct, the clinician instructs the child and consults with the family concerning therapeutic approaches, activities, and implementation of extra-clinic procedures and homework activities. The importance of parents in monitoring changes in the child's stuttering as a result of therapy is stressed more strongly when children are more likely to continue to stutter. In addition, we tend to intensify the involvement of parents and the amount of homework assigned more rapidly with children who are at risk and thus deserve a heightened level of concern.

b. Role of Parents. As stated previously, parental roles are central when children are at risk for continued stuttering. Our rationale is that parents spend more time with their child and are therefore the most important "players," as well as "experts," when it comes to their child, their child's stuttering, and his or her response to indirect and/or direct therapy techniques. In particular, we want parents to stress the importance of communicating to their children, regardless if the output is fluent. It is imperative that parents avoid becoming "The Stuttering Police," as our colleague, Bill Murphy, calls it, and instead focus on encouraging their child to talk whenever, about whatever, and to whomever they choose—bumps, sticky stuff, and all!

c. Role of Others. The roles of others in the lives of children at risk for chronic stuttering are the same as those described for children whose stuttering is likely to be temporary. We rely heavily on parents to familiarize us with their child's daily schedule and the important persons and settings their child encounters. However, unlike therapy with children likely to recover, we pursue the additional involvement of people other than parents more aggressively with children whose risk for continued stuttering is greater. This includes direct contact between the child's relatives, teachers, babysitters, daycare workers, and ourselves as is appropriate to the child's needs.

A variety of goals are inherent in the involvement of important listeners in each child's environment. Most basically, our goal is to provide *information* about fluency and stuttering and *suggestions* for maximizing each child's fluency and communication ease and enjoyment. In doing so, our focus is on ensuring that children are encouraged to talk and perceive others in their own environment as accepting and approving of them. Another goal is to provide children with speaking opportunities during which their communicative partners are employing indirect strategies (i.e., reduced rates, increased pauses, reduced talking and/or questioning, good eye contact) that will make it easier for the children to talk. We also seek to provide and recommend additional contexts in which children may practice new skills (such as the use of turtle talk or stretchy speech), thereby maximizing carryover outside the clinic. When children practice their skills outside of therapy, we stress to them (and sometimes their parents) their role(s) as "expert," with listeners following their lead and thus reinforcing each child's knowledge and efforts.

III. THERAPY TECHNIQUES FOR THE PRESCHOOL CHILD

A. Changing Behaviors

The term *behaviors* refers here to the speech and nonspeech behaviors that children who are stuttering produce. These include SLDs as well as the associated physical concomitants (eye blinking, head movement, and so forth) that are representative of stuttering. It is important to note that we do not address nonspeech behaviors directly. It has been our experience that once SLDs and the tension associated with them decrease, nonspeech behaviors are extinguished. Thus, in describing the techniques used to change behaviors, we focus on changing speech behaviors and any emotional or attitudinal reactions children may have to stuttering.

1. Concepts. We have been strongly influenced by our mentor, Dr. Edward G. Conture, in the development of techniques for addressing stuttering in young children. As Conture (1990, 2001) points out, there are two "elements of speech production" that need to be addressed in order for anyone who stutters to be more fluent. These are time and tension.

a. Time. Time is an important aspect of communication for all of us, regardless of age or fluency status. When we are pressured (whether actual or perceived) to talk quickly, we often have both physical and emotional reactions to that pressure. For example, when interacting with someone who frequently interrupts us or breaks eye contact when we are talking, we often try to talk faster and, sensing the impatience of the listener, feel anxious as we struggle to say more in less time. Young children, whose speech, language, motor, and fluency skills are "under construction," may also sense that they are being rushed or that their ability to talk is not in keeping with that of their conversational partner (which may be true). They may try to increase their speech rates, overlap other speakers to finish what they are saying, and/or increase volume in an attempt to hold the conversational floor. In very young children (i.e., 2- to 3-year-olds), pragmatic skills are not sufficiently developed for understanding of appropriate turn-taking behavior and of waiting to talk (or to do anything else). Thus, they may exhibit self-imposed time urgency as they attempt to gain the attention of adult listeners who are otherwise engaged (e.g., talking on the phone, conversing with another adult, caring for another child).

Our purposes for addressing the concept of time include the need to minimize time urgency imposed by the communicative behavior of listeners as well as that created by young children themselves. Variables that are typically targeted for these purposes include speech rate and turn-taking (i.e., pausing between speaking turns; simultalk, particularly that of an interruptive nature; and balancing the frequency and duration of speaking turns).

(1) Speech rate. A focus on speech rate includes attention to the overall rate of speaking of each person as well as the similarities and differences between the rates of conversational partners. This is called dyadic rate. A speaker's overall rate is typically compared with that of others of the same age. Dyadic rate is a comparison of the rates of two speakers in a conversation. For example, to compare the rate of a child with that of an adult conversational partner, we subtract the child's rate from the adult's rate. The larger the difference, the greater the disparity between the adult model and the child's production. Results of several studies have suggested that reductions in the gap between adult and child speech rates may facilitate fluency in some children who stutter (e.g., Kelly, in review; Stephenson-Opsal & Bernstein-Ratner, 1988; Zebrowski, Weiss, Savelkoul, & Hammer, 1996).

(2) Turn-taking. Aspects of turn-taking in conversation may also affect communicative time pressure. These include the frequency and duration of pauses taken by each speaker within his or her conversational turn as well as between turns by different speakers. How long speakers wait to allow others to finish before commencing their own turns, called wait time or turn-switching pause time, may influence the time urgency felt by conversational partners. The frequency and type of simultaneous talking or "simultalk" by speakers is also an important consideration, particularly if the simultalk is interruptive. This occurs when the simultalk results in the abandonment of a speaking turn by the person who was interrupted. The concern, of course, is that children who are frequently interrupted will relinquish the speaking floor rather than attempt to compete for talking time. Research has suggested a possible association between the duration of parental simultalk and the severity of children's stuttering (e.g., Kelly, 1994; Kelly & Conture, 1992).

b. Tension. The concept of tension, when applied to speech behavior, refers to the extra muscular effort that is expended during production of a sound, syllable, or word by a child who is stuttering. Extra tension or effort may occur as a child attempts to push out a sound that does not seem to be coming out by itself. Tension may increase at any level of the speech sound–production system, but it occurs most frequently at the articulatory (e.g., lips pressed together) or phonatory (e.g., abrupt start to a vowel) level. General tension throughout the body, or various parts therein, is also possible, particularly for those children who are surprised or frustrated by their inability to talk and/or are responding to communicative time pressure.

2. Teaching the Skills.

a. Indirect strategies. When using indirect therapy techniques with preschoolers, parents are the primary focus of our teaching, while children receive the benefits of our models and, more importantly, those of their parents. As stated, parents help to identify and then modify any conversational strategies they may be using that may impact their child's fluency. In many cases, parents will identify attributes of their child's stuttering (e.g., stutters more when he or she interrupts me or when excited or tired) which suggest a starting place for indirect treatment. In general, children stutter more when they are having difficulty getting into or competing in conversation and/or are influenced by the excitement, fear, and/or overwhelming nature of a situation. Frequently, parents report that their children stutter less when they are talking or playing one on one with no distractions and during an activity that the child finds enjoyable (e.g., looking at a picture book), but not overly taxing, competitive, or exciting.

Provision of this information paves the way for discussion of conversational dynamics and their natural influence on communicative time pressure, as well as the unique challenges faced by young children who are developing speech, language, motor, cognitive, and psychosocial skills simultaneously and asynchronously. Suggestions are then made for decreasing communicative time pressure for their child during this period of increased stuttering. Suggestions include decreasing overall rate of speech, enhancing turn-taking ease by pausing longer, and avoiding interruptive simultalk. For some children, having more opportunities to hold the conversational floor is also fluency-facilitating. For other children, the more they talk, the more they stutter (Kelly, in review).

(1) Reducing speech rate. There are many methods that may be used to teach parents to decrease their speech rates. In our experience, it is easier for most adults to add longer pauses between phrases and sentences than to try to produce words at a slower rate (i.e., silence is easier to manipulate than speech). Therefore, we ask parents to try pausing between phrases and sentences, first during reading and then during conversational speech, in interaction with us and by following our models. We then ask them to continue to do so in the presence of both the clinician and their child. Once they feel comfortable with rate reduction, we observe them in interaction with their child alone, provide feedback, and then discuss appropriate times and situations for them to implement reduced speech rate outside of the clinic.

Several questions typically arise concerning this technique, including "How slow is slow enough?" and "How often must we implement this technique with our children?" Although research has not yet suggested an ideal rate for parents to produce in interaction with their preschoolers who are stuttering, it is our experience that a rate within 20 to 30 syllables per minute (spm) of their child's rate is ideal. Depending on how much of a change this will demand for a particular parent, smaller approximations to the target may be taken at first and gradually extended. We also rely on parents to communicate their own comfort levels with incremental changes in their speech rates.

Some parents tell us that they will implement the decreased rate in every situation beginning immediately. These are typically well-meaning parents who want to make sure that we understand their high level of commitment to helping their child. In addition, they have had little experience with modifying their natural speech rates and are, therefore, sometimes overly optimistic about their abilities to, and tolerance for, implementing this change. We typically respond by letting them know that rate is not something that is easy to change because of its signature quality. In other words, we each speak at a rate that is natural for us physically, emotionally, and pragmatically. We also stress the need to start small and achieve accuracy before attempting to generalize to additional situations. Sometimes, we provide analogies to learning other skills, like playing musical instruments or sports. When mastering such skills, brief daily periods of practice are more fruitful than protracted intense practice periods all at one time. Parents are asked to help us determine the best days, times, and contexts to begin to implement change.

(2) Increase duration of turn-taking pauses. Another change we ask parents to make tends to be easier than reduction of speech rate. If parents are having difficulty with rate reduction and/or evince frequent interruptive simultalk in interaction with their child, we suggest focusing on turn-taking. Most simply, we ask parents to count, "a-one and a-two" (with all due thanks to Lawrence Welk), before responding to a comment or question by their child. At times, if the child is excited and/or desires a quick re-

sponse, he or she may resume talking before the parent has a chance to respond. However, if the child truly wants an answer or response, he or she will eventually wait and listen. If the child is old enough and understands the concept, parents may implement a turn-taking rule or signal (e.g., holding up a hand to indicate "wait") when the child (or another family member) fails to pause for a requested response or for completion of another's turn. With children under 4 years of age, a concrete signal may be necessary, at least initially, to teach the concept of turn-taking. In group therapy with preschoolers, we use something visible and tangible like a turtle puppet, talking wand, or a hand signal (e.g., raising) to identify the individual whose turn it is to speak. With very young children (i.e., 2- to 3-year-olds), we may begin by placing them in a line and giving them speaking turns only when they are at the head of the line. Additional cues (e.g., green circles for "go" and red circles for "stop") may also be used.

When parents and/or children tend to talk simultaneously, particularly when it results in the abandonment of a turn by the original speaker, we advise parents to make an attempt to end all unnecessary interruptions. Implementation of increased pausing, as described above, usually takes care of this. However, in some situations, parents (or siblings or others in the child's environment) will jump in and finish what the child is saying, typically because they know what the child is going to say and want to be helpful when the child is stuck (or taking too long to talk). As with simultalk, we ask parents (and other listeners) to eliminate this behavior, waiting patiently until the child finishes. This makes some adults uncomfortable, because it is difficult to watch a young child struggle while speaking, and they want to help. In response to this, we suggest that parents feel free to acknowledge the difficulty the child just experienced and compliment the content of the child's utterance by saying, for example, "That was a little hard for you to say, wasn't it? That's okay. I'm listening, and I really like all the wonderful things you have to tell me."

b. Direct strategies. When using direct therapy techniques, the child learns ways to decrease time pressure and physical tension. These include reducing speech rate through the use of turtle speech (the first level of direct treatment); contrasting easy versus hard or sticky versus smooth speech (second level); and preventing or modifying stuttering by use of stretchy (i.e., prolonged) speech and/or soft touches (i.e., light articulatory contacts) (third level).

(1) Turtle speech. At the first level of direct therapy, we begin by contrasting the concepts of *fast* and *slow*. We contrast walking, running, skipping, coloring, bicycling, and performing other fine and gross motor tasks at fast and slow rates. We emphasize how one is more likely to lose control when performing any of these skills too quickly. We demonstrate ourselves, have children practice, and play with animal and human figurines to contrast fast (out of control) with slow (in control) movements.

We read or paraphrase the classic Aesop fable, *The Tortoise and the Hare*, and talk about why the tortoise won the race. We have found the illustrated version for 4- to 8-year-olds to be particularly useful for our preschoolers who stutter (Granowsky, Cartier, & Bettoli, 1996). We then introduce fast and slow talking. The model for fast talking is a rabbit that has trouble being understood and runs out of breath as a result of trying to get everything out so quickly. In contrast, the turtle is introduced as the slow-talking model. He (or she, when the child is female) is calm, cool, and collected and speaks at a rate that is "nice and easy for us to listen to" or is "just right." The rabbit's pace is extremely fast, yet the turtle's pace is not extremely slow; rather, he talks like Mr. Rogers. His rate, as modeled by the SLP, is slowed by the insertion of pauses between phrases, sentences, and before initiating his own speaking turns. Mr. Rabbit then remarks about how wonderful Mr. Turtle's talking sounds are, which is followed by a request for Mr. Turtle to "teach me how to talk like you." We then enlist the child's help (or the help of all the children in a group setting) in teaching Mr. Rabbit how to use turtle speech. We also reinforce the ideas that "it's okay to talk too fast sometimes," and "it takes awhile to learn new things."

(2) Easy versus hard and sticky versus smooth. At the second level of direct therapy, we focus more specifically on ac-

knowledging the fact that speech can be easy and smooth versus hard, sticky, and/or bumpy. Our choice of terms depends on a number of factors. The first is how the child describes his or her own stuttered speech. If the child says it is "hard," we use that term; if "bumpy," then we use that term. If a child is unable to describe what it is like, we demonstrate different types of stuttered speech and see to which terms the child relates best. We then talk about how using turtle speech can help us to keep our speech smooth, and we practice, beginning with words and building to phrases, sentences, picture descriptions, storytelling, and then conversation. We do not typically start with isolated phonemes or syllables, because these units are too brief for adequate practice of turtle speech.

(3) Stretchy speech. If turtle speech is not sufficient to decrease stuttering behavior and, in particular, any tension or struggle apparent during stuttered moments, stretchy speech is recommended. Stretchy speech is the production of slightly prolonged consonants and vowels, particularly at the beginning of the target linguistic unit (i.e., word, phrase, or sentence). With very young children, it is best to start by stretching every single sound. With the use of stretchy hair ties, large elastic bands, taffy, and/or strings of licorice, we model and have the child imitate stretching out sounds, beginning in isolation, then in syllables, and finally in words, stretching them out as long as possible. We challenge the child to see who can stretch a sound for the longest time and who has the best stretches at the syllable and/or word levels. The exaggerated stretching tends to be very fluency facilitating, an effect that is maintained as we gradually decrease the length of the stretch. The end target is the addition of only a brief stretch at the beginning of words, phrases, and then sentences. The elastic bands are faded out and replaced with a gesture (i.e., fingers of both hands pulling away from one another) that is used on occasion to remind the child to add a little stretch (without necessitating an interruption of ongoing speech), and then also faded out.

Another helpful activity is to have the child take turns being the "teacher." Whoever has the role of teacher holds the elastic band and elongates it to indicate to the "student" to add a stretch while talking. This helps to extend the concept to higher levels of production such as full sentences, picture descriptions, storytelling, and conversation. Parents also may be included in this activity with the child as the role of teacher, who models, requests, and then evaluates the parents' success with the technique.

(4) Soft touches. Children tend to increase tension in their articulators or throat when initiating sounds, so we may teach them how to produce light articulatory contacts. These are known as soft or light touches and are introduced at the third level of direct therapy. With preschoolers, this lesson is best taught by initially contrasting hard and soft objects. One technique that has been enjoyable, and successful with many preschoolers is the use of marshmallows, some of which have been left out and allowed to harden and others that have been preserved in their preferred soft and pliable state. We then talk about hard versus soft marshmallows and contrast them with hard versus soft touches (i.e., articulatory contacts). For example, the lips are pressed hard or softly together, and/or pushing out a vowel (while squeezing the marshmallow) versus easing it out (while touching it gently, often with a little stretch). As was the case with stretchy speech, the level of difficulty is gradually increased from isolated sounds to syllables, words, phrases, sentences, and so forth. Case Example 4-9 is a sample activity for teaching preschoolers about the concepts of sticky, bumpy, or hard versus smooth/easy, while employing turtle and/or stretchy speech, as well as soft touches, as indicated by the child's needs and level of therapy.

B. Addressing Emotional Responses

1. **Emotional Reactions of Children Who Stutter.** Many preschoolers who stutter evince few, if any, emotional reactions to stuttering. For these children, we focus on other aspects of the problem and monitor them closely for any changes in emotional reactions. Other preschoolers who stutter may show mild surprise or fleeting frustration with their inability to say what they want to say as quickly and easily as they want to say it. This may be a result of a more general intolerance of making mistakes (see Case Example 4-4) or frustration with a change in speaking proficiency

Case Example 4-9

On the Road

1. Draw or set up objects to form a roadway. Your roadway will need smooth stretches of road and then various obstacles. The obstacles may include railroad tracks, a mud slick or oil spill, a drawbridge, and a closed roadway with a detour.
2. For every obstacle, there should be an alternative path (e.g., a detour) or way to continue moving through the obstacle (e.g., the drawbridge reconnects, the road is repaired).
3. Let the child choose a vehicle and choose a vehicle yourself to go "on the road."
4. Focusing on one SLD at a time, analogize each obstacle on the road to bumpy, hard, or sticky speech and each detour or "repair" to smooth or easy speech. Only include those obstacles that are representative of the child's SLDs. We typically use the following:
   a. railroad tracks: sound/syllable or monosyllabic whole word repetitions (e.g., "Gi-Gi-Gi-Give") = bumpy speech
   b. mud slick or oil spill: audible sound prolongations (e.g., "lllllllllike") = sticky speech
   c. drawbridge: broken words (e.g., "w...hat") = sticky or hard speech
   d. closed roadway: inaudible sound prolongations or silent "blocks" (e.g., "..... I") = sticky or hard speech
5. Negotiate your car around the roadway, modeling the types of SLDs and calling them sticky, bumpy, or hard.
6. Have the child drive his or her car to the appropriate obstacle upon hearing you produce bumpy, sticky, or hard speech. Listen to what the child calls it, and use that terminology in the future. Ask, "What kind of speech was that?"
7. Show the child how you can take the smooth detour around all of the obstacles by using your turtle, smooth, or easy speech techniques. Have the child identify when you take the smooth or easy road and when you take the bumpy, sticky, or hard road. Again, listen to the terms the child uses and adopt them for future activities.

(continues)

(continued)

8. Build from simple to more complex linguistic structures (i.e., words, phrases, sentences, multiple sentences, picture descriptions, stories, conversation).

9. With children at the second level of direct therapy, focus on using turtle speech to stay on the smooth or easy road. Sticky, bumpy, or hard speech is not practiced by the child at this level. Rather, the child recognizes it in your speech and then shows you how to use turtle speech to stay on the smooth road (i.e., to detour around the SLDs).

10. With children at the third level of direct therapy, have them contrast sticky, bumpy, or hard speech with easy or smooth speech, both in your speech and in their own. They may also use (and suggest you use) turtle and/or stretchy speech and/or soft touches to keep speech smooth and easy and proceeding along the detours.

for those who are accustomed to frequent and effortless communication. A few children who stutter, especially those with more sensitive temperaments, may become quite upset about their stuttering—crying, voicing frustration, and/or refusing to talk. When asked, they may admit that their speaking difficulties make them "sad," "mad," or even "scared."

If a child shows surprise or frustration with so-called mistakes made while talking, we focus on helping the child to understand and accept that we all make mistakes when we are learning to talk (or walk, color, read, and so forth). We emphasize the content of the child's message (i.e., knowledge, ideas, imagination) as more important than the manner in which it is produced (i.e., fluent or disfluent). It is also helpful to acknowledge the child's surprise and/or frustration calmly and directly with responses such as, "That was a little hard to say, wasn't it? That's okay. Everyone gets stuck sometimes. I like all the wonderful things you tell me!" These responses may be modeled for and implemented by parents. Just as we acknowledge a child's bruised knee with calm and compassion, we may acknowledge the "bumps" and "scrapes" that children encounter when talking. It is always better to acknowledge the child's emotional response and provide comfort than to ignore the difficulties with silence. Offering consolation and acceptance, using words as well as actions (e.g., a touch, smile, hug), will put both the child and the listener at ease. The trick, as with bruised knees, is to respond in a manner and to a degree appropriate to the child's own response and emotional state.

2. **Emotional Reactions of Parents of Children Who Stutter.** In our experience, parents may respond nonverbally, indicating surprise, frustration, or fear, without even knowing their responses are perceptible. They may look away from the child or at one another in silence, afraid to say anything, assuming that a verbal response will draw the child's attention to the stuttering and thus make it worse. When discussing their child's stuttering, some parents tell us that it makes them sad, angry, afraid, ashamed, worried, and/or frustrated. Such feelings are often the result of the helplessness they feel when their child stutters. They are not sure what to say or do, whether the stuttering is normal or abnormal, and, most of all, have no idea how to help their child.

When working with parents who are reacting emotionally to their child's stuttering, we begin by providing reassurance and then help them to provide the same for their child. As Dean Williams (1982) suggested, we help them to adopt a "calmness that is contagious." We do this by reassuring them that they are not to blame; that their feelings are natural and stem from the love, care, and concern they have for their child; and that there are ways to help their child. The first step for parents is to *reassure* their children that they love them, enjoy communicating with them, and understand their frustration when talking. We help the parents to *focus* on the positives about their child and the child's communication, and encourage the parents to *bind* their feelings with constructive activities (e.g., spending one-on-one relaxed interaction times with their child, tracking their child's stuttering, and observing their child during daily activities) (Schum, 1986).

3. **Attitudinal Responses of Children Who Stutter.** On occasion, we have worked with preschoolers who are afraid to talk because they might stutter. Upon closer examination, we often discover that these children are concerned that the problem may not go away or may even get worse, making them unable to talk at all. Some children may also have hypotheses or theories about why they stutter. Case Example 4-10 explains one child's theory about her stuttering.

Case Example 4-10

During Mandi's initial evaluation, her SLP asked her why she thinks she sometimes has trouble talking. Mandi reported that it all started after she used baby talk (repetitions of sounds and syllables: "googoo," "baba," etc.) one day. She said that she had been talking like a baby, went to sleep that night, and the next morning she sounded just like a baby whenever she talked. No matter what she tried, she couldn't seem to change it.

Once again, respond to these reactions with calmness and reassurance. Let children know they can learn easier ways of talking—an offer that is typically met with relief and an eagerness to learn.

Other children who stutter may respond in ways that indicate they have adopted the attitudes and/or reactions of their parents. One way we discern a child's reaction to stuttering is to watch and listen to the child's responses to our "pretend" stuttering. We typically model stuttering that is similar to that produced by the child, without it being extremely long, tense, or exacerbated. Case Example 4-11 illustrates this technique and a child's adoption of his father's attitude as expressed during his initial evaluation.

Case Example 4-11

When interacting with Louis, the SLP commented, "I c-c-can get there first. Hmm, I got a little stuck there. Does that ever happen to you?" Before she finished her question, Louis said, "N-n-no, you can't do that. That's not good. That's bad. You can't go 'c-c-c' like that." The SLP commented, "I can't. Why not, Louis?" Louis responded, "Cuz Daddy said it not good to go c-c-c like that. It bad. You gotta stop that and talk good." The SLP replied that she sometimes has trouble talking, and Louis said, "Me too." The SLP then commented, "That's okay. We all get stuck sometimes."

Case Example 4-11 reflects an attitude held by a parent and communicated clearly to the child who passed the advice along to the SLP. When stuttering is seen as bad, wrong, or unacceptable, children are more likely to see their talking as flawed and potentially avoid stuttering and even talking itself. This may lead to increasingly negative attitudes and feelings about stuttering, speaking, communicating, and, in some children, a generally negative attitude about themselves. It is important that we address these attitudes when they are revealed by the child, as well as help parents to recognize the impact of their verbal and nonverbal responses on their child's speaking and self-perceptions. We must help children to "develop constructive beliefs about and realistic perceptions of themselves and of the talking that they do" (Williams, 1982, p. 60).

4. **Attitudinal Responses of Parents of Children Who Stutter.**
   Case Example 4-11 illustrates a hazard of negative parental attitudes about stuttering. The reactions to stuttering by parents (and other significant persons in the child's environment) influence the child's viewpoints about stuttering. Parents may respond nonverbally—frowning, tensing, or looking away—when their child stutters, or they may respond verbally with advice or suggestions for eliminating the stuttering (e.g., "Stop stuttering" or "Slow down" or "Think about what you're saying" and/or "Stop and start over"). In response, children may attempt to implement their parents' specific suggestions or may make changes on their own in an effort to hide or disguise the behavior that is unacceptable to their parents. Unfortunately, the advice parents give, while seemingly logical, is often impossible for children to implement, particularly when it is given quickly with obvious frustration and interrupts the child's own attempts to communicate. We like to talk with parents about stuttering in young children as "mistakes made while talking," much like coloring outside the lines is a mistake made while coloring, which are expected during development (Williams, 1982).

Mistakes are expected and are part of the learning process when children are developing numerous skills and abilities in early childhood. If we react to such mistakes as unacceptable, then the child learns that they are unacceptable. If, however, we respond with acceptance and encouragement, then the child learns that the content of his or her communication is much more important than the manner (i.e., the fluency) in which it is produced (Conture,

2001). Helping parents to recognize and eliminate negative reactions, while developing and increasing positive reactions to the child's communicative efforts, gives them opportunities to help that are constructive and foster healthy attitudes about communication and about self in their child.

IV. CONCLUSION

We hope we have illustrated in this chapter that treatment of preschoolers who stutter necessitates thorough examination and consideration of chronicity risk factors, changes in stuttering behavior, the influence of children's development and their environment, and the general progression of the disorder (and other skills and abilities) over time. Related to these aspects, the interplay of behavioral, emotional, and attitudinal components must be carefully considered. By conducting thorough initial and ongoing evaluations of these factors, carefully tracking the child's progression over time, and tailoring our treatment goals and plans to the individual child and family, we are able to achieve substantial success in the remediation of stuttering in preschoolers.

C H A P T E R

5

Therapy for the Elementary School-Age Child

I. EXAMINING THE EVIDENCE

Chapter 4 focused on preschoolers who stutter and for whom stuttering may or may not become chronic. The information provided in that chapter may also be applied to some kindergartners and, on occasion, first or second graders if stuttering has begun recently (i.e., in the past year) and few of the risks of chronic stuttering are present. The children who are the focus of this chapter are those who have been stuttering longer (i.e., more than 12 to 24 months) and are at greater risk for continuing to stutter. These are children for whom a "wait and see" attitude and/or a focus on indirect forms of treatment alone are contraindicated. Thus, a more aggressive approach to therapy is recommended in which speech and nonspeech behaviors, feelings/emotions, and thoughts/attitudes are evaluated and addressed, on a case-by-case basis, beginning as soon as possible, and in an integrated fashion.

A. Results of Assessment

As outlined in Chapter 2, a thorough understanding of the child's stuttering, as well as his reactions to it and those of others, is obtained during the diagnostic process. Frequency, type, and duration of stuttering and nonspeech behaviors associated with stuttering have been identified. The child and the parents have provided information about the consistency and variability of stuttering within and outside of the clinic during interviews and based on data obtained from the parents (and potentially others in the environment, such as teachers). The child has been interviewed regarding personal thoughts and feelings about stuttering and, depending on the age, has completed an instrument such as the Communications Attitudes Test—Revised (DeNil & Brutten, 1991). Parents' (non)verbal behaviors, interaction styles, attitudes, and feelings about stuttering have also been tapped through observations and interviews. Using this information, we evaluate the extent to which speech behaviors, attitudes, and emotions of the child, and responses to and feelings about stuttering by the parent(s) (and others such as teacher, peers, siblings, etc.), appear to be important to the treatment of stuttering for a particular child.

B. Weighing the Factors

Development of a treatment plan for the school-age child who stutters is dependent upon a number of factors, including: (1) behavioral, emotional, and attitudinal components; (2) therapy setting; (3) participants; and (4) approaches to therapy. We contend that the first factor (the components of stuttering) influences decisions made about the others, and emotions and attitudes determine the extent to which behavioral change is possible, particularly outside of the therapy setting.

Speech behavior, or the stuttering itself, is often the easiest to change. Most children, even when stuttering is frequent and severe, can learn one or more techniques for modifying stuttered moments or producing fluent speech with the help of a clinician. Instructions and task difficulty may be adjusted to ensure success with various techniques for facilitating fluency. Children typically become very fluent in the controlled, safe, and supportive therapy environment. If, however, our assessment reveals that the child has negative self-perceptions (in general and/or in relation to stuttering), fears about speaking and/or stuttering, and/or avoids communicating because of stuttering and/or others' reactions to it, generalization to environments outside of the safe, supportive clinical setting may not occur. Children with negative attitudes and/or emotions are less likely to engage in communication; implement their new skills; or change their previous patterns of interaction (e.g., avoiding persons, situations, words) without direct attention to these factors within and outside of therapy. Thus, as will be detailed later in this chapter, the presence of negative attitudes and emotions concerning speech, self, or communication in general will be weighted more heavily in those children who evidence them, because their effects on therapeutic success are manifold.

In addition to examining the child's stuttering and related attitudes and emotions, we also examine the behaviors, attitudes, and emotions of the parents and others in the child's environment as we develop the treatment plan. Looking beyond the child to the environment in which he or she lives is critical to treating stuttering. As suggested previously, increased fluency in the therapy setting does not quickly or easily translate to fluency outside of therapy when the child or significant others have fears, negative attitudes and perceptions, or behaviors that may prevent the child from succeeding in utilizing therapeutic tools in daily living. The experience of gaining control over one's speaking abilities may positively affect the attitudes, feelings, and reactions of the child and of others, as many proponents of "fluency shaping" approaches to treatment propose. However, depending on the duration and pervasiveness of emotional and/or attitudinal overlays, success may be limited. Another concern directly related to others in the child's environment is the frequent expectation that the child's abilities to use fluency-facilitating strategies in the clinic can and should translate into their use outside of the clinic on a consistent basis. It is imperative that we use our objective data and the subjective observations of the child, parents, and others to estimate the relative weight of various factors in the child's stuttering problem.

Figure 5.1 illustrates three hypothetical children and the relative contributions of behavioral, emotional, and attitudinal components to their stuttering problems. Child 1 exhibits a fairly equal balance between behavioral, emotional, and attitudinal components. For this child, the three aspects interact, but none outweighs the others in focus or impact. Thus, the treatment plan will attend equally to all three factors. The stuttering profile for Child 2 is weighted more heavily for speech behavior. This may indicate that the child has a stuttering problem that is more complex and/or severe in terms of the speech behavior he or she produces (e.g., long, tense blocks; multiple iterations of sounds; frequent secondary behaviors), but attitudes and/or behaviors are positive and nonavoidant of stuttering and/or communication. This child may be evidencing complex

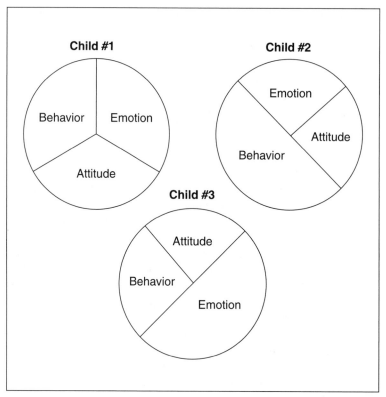

FIGURE 5.1   Hypothetical profiles weighing behavioral, emotional, and attitudinal contributions to stuttering.

patterns of stuttering and may have concerns concomitant to stuttering (e.g., phonological and/or language delay or disorder). Emotional and attitudinal components, while present, are less influential and pervasive in Child 2's stuttering profile. Child 3 has a much more pronounced emotional component to his or her stuttering. This child may possess a sensitive temperament and/or an external locus of control that contributes to feelings of guilt, shame, helplessness, and inadequacy as a speaker. The stuttering may not be as severe or as pervasive as in other children (e.g., Child 2), but the child is emotionally upset by its presence.

The three case examples have been presented in simplified form to provide a starting point for discussing the importance of focusing holistically on each child's stuttering profile. In the following section, we will elaborate on each of the three factors and their potential contributions to stuttering, as well as the impact that the child's environment (e.g., home, school, social) may have.

II. DEVELOPING THE TREATMENT PLAN

A. Considerations

First we consider the relative contributions of behavioral, emotional, and attitudinal components to stuttering in each of our clients. This will determine the types of goals we set and the order in which we address them. As we specify our treatment goals, we must also consider the setting(s) in which therapy will be provided; the composition of the therapy "team" (i.e., the participants in the therapeutic process); and the type of approach we will take. Each of these is considered in more detail below.

1. **Behavioral, Emotional, and Attitudinal Components.** As illustrated in Figure 5.1, three major factors warrant consideration in developing treatment plans. The choice of these three factors or components is not new to literature on stuttering treatment. They are often referred to as the "ABCs" of stuttering (e.g., Cooper & Cooper, 1995; Siegel, 1999). The A stands for affective (i.e., emotional), B for behavioral, and C for cognitive (i.e., attitudinal). Thus, the ABCs of stuttering, or similar terms, could be used interchangeably with those presented in Figure 5.1.

2. **Setting.** In recent years, a number of developments in the field of speech-language pathology have occurred that are both exciting and conducive to improved therapeutic practice regarding persons with communicative disorders. Speech-language pathologists are increasingly working, not only in their own employment facilities, but also in other settings such as clients' homes, school classrooms, and daycare/after-school-care facilities, and in collaboration with other professionals across treatment settings (Zebrowski & Cilek, 1997). These types of joint or collaborative efforts are needed to address natural variations in stuttering and challenges posed by different settings and communication partners for clients to be successful in treatment.

3. **Participants.** When therapy is collaborative and implemented across settings, it will involve a variety of people, the first being the school-age child who stutters. Other participants include the child's parents, siblings, peers, teachers, and additional professionals (e.g., SLPs in other settings, daycare personnel, coaches, grandparents). The more inclusive we are of the settings and persons with whom the child interacts, the more likely we are to develop a treatment plan that positively affects every facet of the

child's daily communication. Such inclusiveness, however, comes at a price. The number of participants and the variety of settings can become exponentially large, making coordination difficult. Later in this chapter we provide some suggestions for making inclusiveness work, including methods for communication among team members (e.g., notebooks, conferences, phone calls, e-mail, reports); for emphasizing the role of the child as the team leader; and for developing a therapy plan that addresses goals, settings, participants, and selected approaches to therapy.

4. **Approach.** If we return to Figure 5.1, we see that Child 2, for whom behavior is the main concern, may benefit most from a fluency shaping (FS) approach that focuses on equipping him or her with tools for producing fluent speech (e.g., reduced rate, prolonged speech, reduced tension in the speech production apparatus) and inclusion of stuttering modification (SM) techniques, as needed, to address attitudes and/or emotions that may surface during treatment, particularly as gains in therapy are transferred outside of the clinical setting.

   Child 3, for whom the emotional component is most prevalent, may be best served by a SM approach in which feelings about oneself— as a person, as someone who stutters, and/or as a communicator— are the principal focus. Discussions and exercises focusing on uncovering, acknowledging, understanding, and changing feelings are highlighted. Speech behavior will also be addressed to help the child gain tools for changing the way he or she speaks and/or stutters so that the "new way of talking" can be applied to situations in which negative feelings have been addressed. As feelings become more positive and the child begins to gain confidence as a speaker, attitudes are also likely to change, and will be addressed as needed.

   Child 1 exhibits equal contributions of behavioral, emotional, and attitudinal components. Thus, development of the treatment plan will focus on addressing each of these simultaneously. From our perspective, this typically involves a combination of FS and SM procedures in which the issues of "how we talk" (i.e., speech behaviors), "how we feel about talking," and "what we think about talking" are addressed.

   An integrated approach to fluency therapy, as illustrated, requires careful attention to the relative contributions of behaviors, emotions, and attitudes to stuttering for each child who stutters. By carefully evaluating and delineating the specific evidence that contributed to the relative weighting of factors we have determined, we may then identify specific treatment objectives, techniques, and the role of each person on the therapy team for the school-age child who stutters.

B. Treatment Objectives

Treatment objectives are the who, what, when, where, why, and how of stuttering intervention. Specifically, "who" refers to the individuals who will be included in each objective; "what," to the short- or long-term goals identified and in what order they will be addressed; "when," to the timing of each objective in the treatment plan; "where," to the context in which each objective will be carried out; "why," to the rationale for each objective; and "how," to the manner in which progress will be evaluated. By attending to each of these questions, we are able to develop a clear treatment plan, both at the beginning of therapy and at each juncture along the way (i.e., daily, weekly, monthly).

A critical element in the development of a treatment plan is the understanding and delineation of the roles of the team members involved in each child's therapy. We believe that by maintaining a primary focus on the people, rather than on the armamentarium of therapy techniques, positive, realistic, and long-term change may be accomplished that is meaningful and positive for all concerned, particularly the child who stutters. In addition, a focus on the person typically yields the type of client-clinician relationship and necessary rapport to help clients (and clinicians) to hang in there over the long road, negotiating all the bumps along the way (e.g., Schum, 1986; Zebrowski & Schum, 1993).

1. **Child's Role.** We begin with the role of school-age children, because they are the primary focus of our therapeutic interactions. Their perspective serves as the starting point for every step in the clinical process. During our initial evaluations, we have tapped their behaviors, feelings, and attitudes about stuttering to give us an idea of where they are in the development of stuttering; how it has affected, and is affected by, their way of perceiving the world, themselves, others, and the stuttering itself; and what they think does and does not help. We begin by using language that focuses on the child as the "quarterback," "director," and/or "expert." Although the clinicians know a lot about stuttering in general, the child knows everything there is to know about his or her own

stuttering. Thus, therapy cannot and will not be successful without the client playing the lead role. Although probably an overused term in any type of counseling, whether for communication disorders or otherwise, it is true that the child must be *empowered* to be in charge when it comes to treating the stuttering (e.g., Luterman, 1996). The use of analogies, such as those stated or alluded to here (e.g., driver, director, lead actor, quarterback, expert) is very helpful in *enabling* (another oft-used counseling term) the client to assume a role in therapy. By getting to know the children and learning what is important, enjoyable, and motivating for them, clinicians can select analogies, terminology, and activities that fit their needs.

2. **Clinician's Role.** As professionals, we have a tendency to let our expertise take precedence over whatever ideas, perceptions, and/or feelings our clients disclose, no matter what their age. We want to take charge and lead our clients wherever we want them to go; however, as the old saying goes, "You can lead a horse to water, but you can't make it drink." As Schum (1986; and Zebrowski & Schum, 1993) emphasize, this type of approach places us in the role of "sage on the stage," and minimizes the client's input, participation, and responsibility for the problem and its solution. In contrast, if we see ourselves as the coach on the sidelines (Schum, 1986), or as a teammate (particularly for those children who initially shy away from leadership roles), then the focus remains on the perspective, needs, abilities, and accomplishments of the child. We must provide the framework or boundaries in which therapy will take place. This necessitates a thorough, up-to-date understanding of stuttering; a careful and comprehensive evaluation; and careful planning, implementation, and documentation of therapeutic objectives, procedures, and results.

3. **Parental Role(s).** The role of parents in stuttering therapy with school-age children changes with the age of the child, as well as with the dynamics of the family. The older the child, the more critical the child's input when deciding how, when, and where to include one or both parents. In our experience, putting parents in the role of clinician, teacher, or sage, when it comes to changing stuttering, is contraindicated, particularly with older school-age children. We do not want to put parents in the position of having to evaluate and/or correct their child's stuttering or use of techniques. Parents have enough teaching and guiding to do in their roles as

parents. They are not experts in stuttering, and we should not expect that of them. In some cases, children will even comment to their parents, "You are not my teacher." Parents are, for obvious reasons, less than objective when it comes to their children and their children's stuttering. This may be particularly problematic when there is a prior history of stuttering in the family; perhaps even the parents themselves stutter. Case Examples 5-1 and 5-2 illustrate these points. Case Example 5-1 focuses on a 9-year-old

---

Case Example 5-1

Mr. and Mrs. S. had, together or individually, watched their 11-year-old son, Tim, in therapy for many months. They were pleased and excited to see his progress. They had participated in Tim's therapy sessions in the clinic and helped him with his "speech homework" when asked by Tim at home.

In the clinic, and when speaking one-on-one to family members or friends, Tim was fluent. When faced with more challenging situations in the clinic (e.g., making phone calls, introducing himself to strangers, competing in a game requiring rapid verbal responses), Tim used brief stretches (i.e., prolongations of initial sounds of phrases) to help him maintain fluency. He reported that he had begun talking more often outside of the clinic and his home, especially at school.

Tim's parents noted that he continued to stutter, and would often increase his rate and exhibit tension in his face and neck when speaking with several family members simultaneously (e.g., at the dinner table), when playing excitedly with his brothers, and/or when speaking with new people. They lamented the fact that "Tim is not using his tools" in these situations. They commented, "We know he can do it. We've seen him use his tools in all kinds of situations in the clinic, even with strangers, on the phone, and with lots of people in the room." They asked the SLP, "Why doesn't he use his tools more often? Is he just being lazy? We remind him, but then he gets upset with us and refuses to talk. We're just trying to help."

(continues)

(continued)

In private, Tim reported that his parents frequently tell him to "just use your tools." He expressed frustration by saying, "They don't care about anything I say, only about whether I stutter or not. I know it embarrasses them, but I can't help it. Sometimes I just want to talk. So what if I stutter."

With the SLP's assistance, Tim had a conversation with his parents in which he talked about the fact that using his tools is not automatic and is hard when he is excited, frustrated, or nervous in a particular situation. He also let them know that he does not want to have to use his tools all the time and that he would like them to try not to remind him to do so. He asked them to continue to practice with him and promised to continue working hard to achieve the goals he set for himself in therapy. Tim's parents reassured him that they are interested in what he has to say, whether he stutters or not, and that they want to help him in any way they are able. They agreed to stop reminding him to use his tools and to continue to participate in activities within and outside of therapy as Tim saw fit. Tim expressed an interest in working with his parents to improve his ability to communicate at the dinner table. Together with the SLP, Tim and his parents decided to "brainstorm" ideas for working on this situation at the next therapy session.

who was making significant gains in therapy but had difficulties in more challenging situations. His parents were confused about the variability in his abilities to use his tools. Case Example 5-2 centers on a family in which a strong history of stuttering was evident on the father's side. The impact of that history on the perceptions and fears of the father of a 7-year-old who stutters is highlighted.

4. **Teacher Role(s).** Teachers play important roles in the lives of school-age children, regardless if they are active participants in fluency therapy programs. The classroom is filled with activities, expectations, interactions, and contexts that challenge intellectual, social, emotional, and verbal skills. The responses of teachers and peers to a child's stuttering may dictate the extent to which the

---

Case Example 5-2

Daniel G., a first grader, was receiving fluency therapy at school twice a week. His mother observed his therapy once a month and spent time with Daniel at home practicing smooth speech while engaged in various activities suggested by the SLP. After 2 months of therapy, Daniel was able to use his smooth speech in a variety of activities that required production of words, phrases, and simple sentences, in the presence of a slow, smooth speech model.

During a parent conference following one of Daniel's sessions, his mother expressed concern that "Daniel's father has a negative attitude about Daniel's stuttering." She said, "He thinks Daniel can stop stuttering anytime he wants to." Mrs. G. reported that Mr. G. stuttered as a young boy but no longer did so. She guessed that Mr. G. "assumes Daniel will do the same thing." Mrs. G. expressed concern that Mr. G. "is giving Daniel the message that he can stop stuttering if he wants to," and commented, "What if he doesn't? Then he'll feel as though he's disappointed his father. I think he already feels that way sometimes."

The SLP asked Mrs. G. to inquire whether Mr. G. might want to attend a parent conference to provide his own insights about Daniel's stuttering. The meeting took place one month later. Mr. G. stated, "I stuttered when I was Daniel's age. I got sick of it, decided I wasn't going to stutter anymore, and that was the end of it. Daniel needs to make that same decision for himself. Until he does, he will continue to stutter." Upon further inquiry, Mr. G. revealed that his own mother stuttered her whole life. He also said that he has a brother who stutters, "but not very badly."

A discussion ensued in which the likelihood of stuttering running in families and variations in severity, duration, and results of therapy were highlighted. Mr. G. was asked to talk about the worst and best scenarios for Daniel if he were to continue to stutter. In the course of the conversation, it was revealed that Mr. G. "hoped to save his son from a lifetime of people laughing and thinking he's stupid because he stutters."

(continues)

(continued)

Accordingly, "My mother was afraid to talk to pretty much everyone except my father and us kids. I don't want Daniel to be like that. It will be harder for him, because he'll need to get a job and survive in this world." Mr. G. also said that his mother never had therapy, but his brother did. Mr. G. said, "I decided to stop stuttering when I saw kids imitating and teasing my brother for having to go to the speech teacher. I don't want Daniel to go through that. I don't know why it worked for me, but I'd like to help Daniel to do the same if I can."

By providing his insights, the father was able to shed further light on the nature and probable causes of his current attitudes and feelings. It also became abundantly clear that his primary concern was to protect Daniel from any negative consequences of stuttering. The SLP then turned the discussion to the parents' hopes for Daniel, the "place" of stuttering in his future, and the objectives and methods of therapy, including how teasing and other possible consequences of stuttering would be addressed. Mr. G. agreed to be involved in therapy "anyway I can to help my son."

child participates, and even learns, in the classroom environment. Their responses will certainly impact the way children who stutter feel about their stuttering, if not their overall communication and self-perceptions. Thus, it is imperative that therapy for stuttering infiltrates the classroom. This is best accomplished with the active knowledge and participation of classroom teachers.

Teachers may be involved in several ways. They may provide observations of the child's fluency within the classroom. The daily stuttering tracking form (see Appendix A), as discussed, may be used for this purpose, as may brief conversations and/or notes shared with the SLP. Teachers may provide indirect speaking models (similar to those suggested for parents in Chapter 4) in interaction with the child who stutters and his or her peers. Classroom guidelines or rules may include requirements for appropriate turn-taking, including "waiting your turn," "listening when others are talking," and/or "no interrupting when another is speaking." Such rules are appropriate for all children, not just those who stutter, and for the classroom atmosphere in general.

More direct participation by teachers may include conferences held between the SLP and teacher or, particularly for older children, between the child and teacher with the SLP present and facilitating interaction as needed. In some cases, teachers may play active roles in therapy when children stutter in the classroom by complimenting their participation, the content of their verbal contributions, their use of techniques, and/or to remind them to implement certain strategies as previously agreed. It is important to emphasize the need for a primary focus on positive, supportive feedback, with a minimal focus on highlighting unwanted speech behavior. When teachers are involved in cueing children who stutter to change the way they are talking, the exact nature, scope, and context of cueing should be clearly delineated and practiced in advance. In addition, a signal by the child to indicate to the teacher that assistance is, or is not, needed at a particular time should also be included.

Finally, teachers should be involved in creating a climate in the classroom that promotes zero tolerance of teasing or any other form of negative treatment of any child, including the child who stutters. Once again, classroom guidelines or rules may prohibit teasing and encourage respect and cooperation among classmates.

If teasing has become an issue for a particular child who stutters, then a classroom discussion may make an important difference. Bill Murphy, from Purdue University, is well known for his classroom presentations in which he and the child who stutters teach the child's classmates and teacher about stuttering and its treatment. They typically start with a discussion of similarities and differences between people, teasing (its sources and consequences), and proper and improper responses to differences and teasing. Classmates then learn what stuttering is, what is known about it, and even how to stutter. The child who stutters, if desired, is given an opportunity to evaluate the skill with which classmates stutter. The same is done for various therapy techniques, and classmates learn what they should do to be helpful when stuttering occurs. Murphy typically ends the presentation by awarding the child who stutters a certificate as the "expert on stuttering," yielding accolades from his or her classmates. Children who stutter determine both the content of the presentation and the extent to which they want to be involved in teaching the class. Results of this technique have included reductions in amounts of teasing, greater comfort levels with stuttering on the part of both teachers and classmates, other children defending the child who stutters in various contexts (e.g., the playground), and positive feelings (e.g., accomplishment, self-esteem, stuttering is no longer a poorly kept or undisclosed secret) on the part of the child who stutters. Initially, some teachers question the idea, because they have not observed teasing in their classroom, or they are afraid that admitting to stuttering will result in poor treatment by other children or embarrassment for the child who stutters. Typically, a conference with the child and/or SLP will alleviate these concerns. An even more powerful ally in these cases is the endorsement of another teacher who has observed the positive effects of a similar presentation.

5. **Roles of Others.** Significant others may be needed on the child's therapy team, including peers, siblings, grandparents, and coaches. The child's best friend and/or a sibling with whom the child feels comfortable sharing stuttering and working on homework assignments may be instrumental. Involvement of a coach or advisor will help to extend therapy goals and accomplishments to contexts outside of the therapy room. Others (e.g., grandparents or other relatives) with whom the child lives and/or spends a significant amount of time may also be important members. The people selected should be those whom the children identify as important participants in their lives. Both those with whom it is easier and harder to talk should be identified and included at appropriate junctures in therapy. Attention to other significant persons will aid in achieving far-reaching and long-lasting treatment effects.

III. THERAPY TECHNIQUES

A. Changing Behavior

As stated earlier, speech behavior is usually the easiest of the three components (i.e., behavioral, emotional, attitudinal) to change. That may be puzzling, because the very problem for people who stutter is a breakdown in speech motor control, directly affecting speech behavior. Let us explain. We are not saying that it is easy for people who stutter to become fluent. The degree of fluency that may be achieved varies from person to person. What we are saying is that the vast majority of people who stutter can learn new ways of talking—of using their respiratory, phonatory, and/or articulatory systems in a manner that is more conducive to fluent speech production. For some, this means spontaneous fluency; for others, controlled fluency; and for still others, acceptable stuttering (e.g., Guitar, 1998). Persons with severe cognitive deficits may be the exception to our claim, although certain methods (e.g., de-layed auditory feedback) may yield some relief (if fluency is indeed a target in their treatment). In general, however, people who stutter have the ability to understand and change the way they talk.

We agree with the oft-made claim that much of stuttering is what people who stutter do when they try not to stutter. Seeing it as something we do, as opposed to something that happens to us, is an important consideration. By helping children who stutter to identify what they do when they stutter and when they do not stutter, to modify speaking and/or stuttering, and then to practice their new skills in increasingly challenging situations helps them to begin to gain control of their speaking and of their stuttering. If, however, negative feelings and/or attitudes about self, communication, and/or stuttering remain, then these new skills may not be practiced, transferred, or habituated. In other words, FS and/or SM techniques may be used in the clinic, and not outside, or only in those situations that the child who stutters does not already avoid. Thus, it is imperative that behaviors, feelings, and attitudes are all addressed in concert. The amount of emphasis varies with the relative contributions of the three factors, as discussed earlier (see Figure 5.1).

We focus now on techniques for changing speech behavior, with the understanding that they are addressed along with feelings and/or attitudes in keeping with each child's stuttering profile and needs.

1. **Identification.** Identifying stuttering is often a starting point for addressing behavioral aspects of this problem. The underlying logic is that children's understanding of what they do when they do and do not stutter will enable them to change it. This step is also informative, in that children's awareness of and willingness to explore their stuttering and fluency yields clues about the types of techniques that might be best to implement. It also provides information about whether emotional and/or attitudinal issues are present that need to be explored before children are ready to confront their stuttering. If attempts to talk about the stuttering are met with a lowered head, averted eyes, and/or obvious discomfort, then the potential interference of negative emotions and/or attitudes may be indicated.

    It is important to point out that most people, no matter how severe their stuttering, are fluent more often than they stutter. Thus, acknowledging the presence of fluency, studying it, and expanding on it is as important as identifying and changing the stuttering it-self. We address this by helping children to understand how and when they do and do not stutter. This approach would be considered part of a SM, rather than a FS, approach to treatment. With a FS approach, the focus would typically begin with modifying the way the child speaks, as will be discussed later. However, when identification is included as the first step, it begins with determining "how and when I stutter."

We typically initiate identification by asking children to demonstrate their own stuttering. When they do so, we praise their modeling and knowledge (i.e., their expertise) about their stuttering. We then ask them to judge our imitations of their stuttering, encouraging them to correct and model for us until we can imitate them accurately. The rationale provided is that "I want to understand how it feels and what it sounds like when you stutter. That will help us to pick the best tools for making changes."

Often, at this point, we add a type of modification technique, asking the child to "freeze and hold" the stuttering, making it as long and/or tense as possible. This may be accompanied by visual cues such as a tight fist or a racecar stuck in the mud, stopped at a wall, or bumping over railroad tracks. We use props that are meaningful to the child and illustrate the types of disfluencies and physical sensations perceived by the child. We then ask the child to release the tension slowly and finish the word (e.g., Guitar, 1999). We talk about the differences between tense and loose speech, sticky and smooth speech, or stuttered and fluent speech. Verbal praise and encouragement are constant, and tangible rewards (e.g., tokens, stickers, a tally of the number of tries) are used according to what motivates the particular child. The focus is on bringing the stuttering out into the open (a type of desensitization) and demonstrating to children that they have the ability to control it. We use reinforcing phrases such as: "You did it." "That was a really good one." "You really held onto that." "That was incredibly smooth." "You're really an expert at this." "You do a great job changing from tense to smooth." "I can tell you can really feel that."

It is also important to discuss "when I stutter" and "when I do not stutter." As mentioned, people who stutter are fluent more often than they stutter. Stuttering is also predictable, occurring at the beginning of phrases, in words, in sounds and words that the child perceives as more difficult (e.g., particular vowels or consonants, his or her name), and in particular situations (e.g., on the telephone, in the classroom, at the dinner table). We discuss these possibilities with the children and find out when they notice stuttering and when they are fluent. This step allows for reinforcement of the concept that fluency does occur and that "I can be fluent." It also contributes to the development of a clear picture of the variations in fluency in the child's daily life that will be developed into a *situational hierarchy* through which the transfer of new ways of talking will be addressed.

Another helpful method for identifying stuttering, particularly for those children who have limited awareness of when they stutter and/or are reluctant to model their own stuttering, is to have them recognize stuttering in the clinician's speech. To begin, the SLP produces instances of stuttering in his or her speech, telling the child, "See if you can catch me producing bumpy speech, a stutter, or sticky speech." The child is asked to raise a hand, point at the SLP, throw a chip into a bucket, or any other useful indicating strategy. The child is then verbally (and sometimes tangibly) reinforced for "catching the stuttering." The SLP may alter the type, length, tension, and other characteristics of the stutters produced, challenging the child to "see if you can catch me this time."

Once children are comfortable and consistent at identifying the SLP's stuttering, they are asked to talk so the SLP can "catch" their stuttering. Depending on their ability, children may be asked to produce some "pretend" stutters or to talk spontaneously. In either case, they are reinforced for stuttering "well." It may then evolve into a game where the SLP and child take turns stuttering and try to be the first to catch the stuttering. This may be done "on-line" (i.e., in live speech) or "off-line" from audio- or videotapes. We often follow this technique with a focus on "freezing and holding" the stutter, thus progressing toward modifying the stuttering behavior.

Some children, regardless of the technique applied, are unable and/or reluctant to identify their own stuttering while they are producing it. For these children, identifying their own stuttering off-line often follows identifying the SLP's stuttering. To facilitate the transition to self-identification, the child should be asked to imitate the SLP's stutterings, conveying the message, albeit indirectly, that "it's okay to stutter." Once children feel comfortable imitating another's stuttering, they are more likely to identify, imitate, and modify their own stuttering.

2. **Modification.** Many different techniques may be used to modify stuttered moments and/or speaking in general. The needs of the particular child are the main consideration in selecting and implementing various techniques. If a FS approach is taken, the focus will be on talking in a smoother, slower, and/or stretchy manner. The new way of talking is used throughout the speech stream, with a focus on maintaining fluency and/or preventing stuttering from occurring. If a SM approach is taken, more attention is paid to changing stuttering to make it smoother, slower, controlled, and/or easier. Techniques may be used prior to, during, and/or following expected stuttered moments. A combination of techniques from FS and SM may be used, as needed, for particular children. We will now present a few techniques from each of the two major approaches. We do so acknowledging that there are multiple writers and practitioners who have developed, implemented, and refined these approaches. Thus, the following represents a blending of ideas from multiple persons and sources as well as our own experiences.

a. Fluency-shaping techniques. These techniques are aimed at achieving and maintaining fluency, thus eliminating stuttering. They typically include attention to one or more speech-production systems (i.e., respiration, phonation, and/or articulation) and to promote the production of easy, effortless speech. The SLP may begin by helping the child to identify "speech helpers" (i.e., lungs, voice box, articulators) using diagrams, models, and tactile cues (e.g., Ramig, 1999). How speech in general, and speech sounds in particular, are produced is emphasized. Several techniques for producing smooth, fluent speech are then introduced.

(1) "Easy onset of phonation" targets voice production. This is particularly helpful for children who produce silent blocks and/or report tension in the chest and/or neck (i.e., laryngeal) area. The SLP models production of a vowel, "turning on the voice" "easily," "softly," and/or "smoothly." Gradual and controlled voice onset is modeled and imitated by the child. An *h* paired with a vowel is often helpful for teaching this skill. After practicing with vowels and *h*+ vowels, practice extends to the onset of words, phrases, sentences, and from known contexts (e.g., pictures) to unknown contexts (e.g., spontaneous conversation or telephone calls).

(2) Light, articulatory contacts focus on placing the articulators together in a soft, light, or gentle manner. Using various consonants, typically beginning with those that are most visible (i.e., m, p, b, f, v), allows light touches to be modeled and practiced. Illustrations, a mirror, a tongue depressor, or other props may be used to facilitate understanding and production of light, articulatory contacts.

(3) Prolonged or stretched speech is probably the most frequently used technique in FS approaches. Children are taught to stretch and/or connect their sounds, words, phrases, and sentences (e.g., Schwartz, 1999). Vowels and continuant consonants are easiest to prolong. Using light articulatory contacts that allow for a brief release of airflow helps to prolong stop consonants when these phonemes pose difficulties for the child who stutters.

(4) Increasing the duration of pauses between phrases, sentences, speaking turns, and sometimes words results in a decreased speaking rate, called just right, slow, or turtle speech. Children are encouraged to "take their time," "set the pace," "keep it slow and steady," and so forth. Rate control is particularly important when children who stutter experience time pressure, whether actual or perceived. By maintaining a slower rate themselves, no matter what others are doing, they can gain a sense of control over their speech and over the flow of conversation. Both pausing and prolonged speech techniques may be used to accomplish rate reduction. As children begin to master this skill in the clinic, we begin to introduce time pressure by increasing our own rate, interrupting them, ignoring them, walking away, and other such obnoxious behaviors. Children are instructed to "hold their own" no matter what we do. Accomplishing this is very rewarding for children who stutter and helps to prepare them for more difficult contexts and listeners.

b. Stuttering modification techniques. These techniques typically focus on changing stuttering after, during, or before the stuttered moment occurs. They also center more on helping the child accept the stuttering and explore any feelings and attitudes associated with stuttering and speaking than on changing the speech behaviors in isolation. The end goal is to enable the child to communicate whenever and wherever desired, regardless if speech is spontaneously fluent, controlled, or contains acceptable stuttering. Van Riper (1973) introduced three techniques for modifying stuttering that we frequently employ with school-age children who stutter. They are taught in the following sequence.

(1) Cancellation. After a stuttering has occurred, the child waits a few seconds and then produces the stutter again, but in an easier manner that is slower and controlled. Another option is to reproduce the stuttered word fluently.

(2) Pull-out. For the second step, children must catch themselves in a moment of stuttering and then produce a pull-out, easing themself out of the stuttering. This step is also typically applied following "freezing and holding," as described previously. The child must not rush through the rest of the word, but produce it slowly and in a controlled manner as when canceling a stuttered moment.

(3) Preparatory set. The final step involves using a preparatory set before attempting production of an upcoming word that the child anticipates will be stuttered. The first sound of the word is begun slowly, smoothly, and easily by using a slower rate and light articulatory contacts. The word is completed in the same way as for pull-outs—in a slow, relaxed, smooth manner.

The combination of techniques just described (i.e., cancellations, pull-outs, and preparatory sets) are applied to achieve easy stuttering, as described by Van Riper (1973, 1974). In brief, easy stuttering is a slower, more relaxed and controlled manner of stuttering and speaking.

We previously described having children imitate the SLP's and/or their own stuttering. This is called voluntary or pseudo stuttering. Both terms imply stuttering "on purpose," or pretending to stutter as a means of understanding, exploring, and disclosing stuttering. Such purposeful stuttering helps to put children in control of their stuttering while also bringing the stuttering out into the open or, in essence, making it a speakable and hearable topic. This process is frequently desensitizing for both the child and the listener, thus "deawfulizing" the stuttering (Murphy, 1999a & b) for all concerned. It is a powerful way of addressing not only speech behavior, but also negative feelings that children who stutter and/or their listeners have about stuttering.

Those techniques may be integrated, as needed, for each child who stutters. The techniques selected will depend upon the age of the child; the stuttering profile; the results of trial therapy conducted to explore the child's abilities, goals, and interests; and the amount and type of progress that is achieved.

B. Changing Emotions/Feelings

No matter how fluently or disfluently children speak, they are not likely to pursue communicative interactions with others if they do not feel good about themselves as speakers. Their emotions or feelings influence their stuttering. Likewise, stuttering influences their emotions and feelings. As noted for preschoolers, some children are intolerant of any mistakes they make, whether in speaking or otherwise. Even disfluencies judged to create a mild or minor problem may be viewed as debilitating by children. As a result, they may feel ashamed, fearful, inferior, flawed, or any number of other emotions. This may lead to avoidance of not only stuttering, but also of communication in general. As fears persist and are reinforced by children's own perceptions, as well as the reactions of others (and their perceptions of others' reactions), fears become more difficult to overcome. Gaining the ability to modify stuttering and/or produce fluent speech may not result in changes in self-perceptions. An additional concern with the presence of negative feelings is the likelihood that these emotions have become generalized to many contexts and may not be entirely apparent to children who stutter. As a result, their expression may be vague, diffuse, and pervasive. It is important for the SLP to begin to explore each child's feelings, unraveling the many layers of reactions, concerns, and relationships that have developed. This may be accomplished through a sequence of steps that are repeated throughout the therapy process.

1. **Identification.** As described for speech behaviors, we often begin by helping children to identify their emotions and feelings. We are not only interested in those feelings that relate to stuttering, but also in conversing with them individually about who they are as a person.

   a. General Feelings. It is helpful to begin by exploring the general feelings of children. To do this, we often talk about different emotions (happiness, sadness, anger, fear, shame, guilt, excitement, confusion, etc.). We talk about their experiences of those emotions in various situations they encounter on a regular basis and in those situations that are less frequent. We acknowledge children's feelings and help them explore and express those thoughts. Although we do not typically label their emotions, we frequently elaborate on the emotions expressed using their own words. It is often helpful if such conversations are taking place while the clinician and a child are engaged in enjoyable activities (e.g., listening to music, coloring, building, playing a board game, taking a walk). In addition to talking, we may have the child draw pictures, keep a diary or journal, and/or read and respond to various stories about children experiencing various emotions. We sometimes ask children to engage in emotional reminiscences in which they recall times in their lives when they were happy, sad, angry, fearful, etc. (e.g., Denham et al., 1997). We may model such reminiscences for them, using brief episodes from our own experiences, particularly those of childhood. During these discussions, we follow the children's lead, reinforcing them for their insights, excellent memory, and helpful descriptions of their experiences. Once again, the child is viewed as the "expert" when it comes to personal experiences and feelings.

b. Stuttering-Related Feelings. In addition to exploring the child's general feelings and emotions, we also focus on those related to talking and stuttering. The Communications Attitude Test—Revised (CAT-R) (DeNil & Brutten, 1991), as mentioned earlier, provides an excellent tool for exploring not only children's attitudes, but also feelings about their communication abilities. Following completion of the CAT-R, we converse with the child about his or her responses. In addition to determining whether a particular item on the CAT-R is true or false for the child, we gauge the importance and pervasiveness of the content of each item for the child. This helps us to understand the significance of a particular concern. For example, if Sam reports, "I am afraid the words won't come out when I talk," we explore how often this occurs and how it makes him feel. We also ask what he does when he is afraid the words come out and whether this works or not.

Another technique we use is to ask children to describe and/or write what typical weekday and weekend days are like for them. Discussion involves the amount, importance, and difficulty of talking at various junctures in the child's daily routine, and feelings about abilities and difficulties with talking and/or stuttering in various situations. Topics of discussion also include favorite and not so favorite talking activities, the reasons behind the child's preferences, and feelings about the various speaking experiences. Children may write their descriptions in a journal or enter them into a computer. Some clients enjoy sending e-mail logs of their thoughts, feelings, observations, accomplishments, and anything else they wish to share. Others have used the daily stuttering tracking form to estimate their stuttering severity and provide comments about their experiences. This is particularly useful for children who are reluctant or are learning to record their experiences in a written form.

c. Situational Hierarchy. These exercises used to tap the child's general feelings and focus on talking and/or stuttering naturally evolve into the development of a situational hierarchy. Situations in which the child communicates are ordered from least to most difficult, according to the child's descriptions. The hierarchy typically starts out with a few general descriptions of situations and gradually expands into a precisely detailed inventory of communicative experiences. We use the hierarchy for several purposes. First, it gives us an idea of what the child's life outside of the therapy context is like from his or her perspective. Does the child talk frequently? When? With whom? Does the child avoid communicating? When? With whom? Second, it helps us to understand how the child feels about talking and/or stuttering and about the role of others in his or her communicative environment. Third, the hierarchy is instrumental in helping the child to practice, generalize, and solidify changes made in therapy. It must be analyzed, reanalyzed, and modified throughout the therapy process. By producing a written record of the hierarchy, it may be used to illustrate progress as well as to select the next target context for remediating stuttering. The complexity of the hierarchy depends upon a number of factors, including the child's age, the number and variety of contexts in which the child communicates, and the extent to which negative emotions have been associated with talking and/or stuttering. Once again, the particular child, the diagnostic profile, and the individual needs must be considered. Case Example 5-3

Case Example 5-3

Situation	Comments	Rank
Talking to mom	She's a good listener. It's okay to stutter with mom except when I'm practicing my speech. Sometimes she reminds me to use my tools.	4
Talking to my father	Dad doesn't talk a lot. We mostly play ball. My stuttering makes him nervous.	8
Talking to my baby brother	This is easy. I never stutter with him, but he's only a baby.	1
Reading aloud	I never stutter when I read by myself or when I read to my baby brother.	2
Talking to my friends	I can talk okay with one friend, but it's hard with lots of kids at once. I'm mostly quiet then.	6
Talking to my teacher	My teacher is really nice, and I like to talk with her. Sometimes she tells the other kids to be quiet when I'm talking, and I get a little embarrassed.	7
Talking on the phone	My parents always want me to talk to grandma on the phone, and I hate it. She always asks me lots of questions.	10

(continues)

(continued)

Situation	Comments	Rank
Answering questions in class	I never raise my hand, even when I know the answer, and I can feel my face get red when my teacher calls on me. Sometimes I talk okay, and sometimes it's awful.	9
Playing baseball	I'm the first baseman, and it's really fun. I don't have any trouble talking, cuz we mostly play.	3
Going to Sunday school	The teacher picks on the kids who don't do their homework, so I make sure mine is done.	5

contains the first draft of a situational hierarchy that was developed by a 9-year-old as a homework assignment. He listed the situations, commented about them, and then ranked them from "easiest" to "hardest." He identified 10 situations, but children may select as many situations as they desire. A blank form of the hierarchy is provided in Appendix C.

2. **Modification.** Negative emotions and feelings that interfere with the child's abilities and/or willingness to communicate must be addressed once they have been uncovered. Without doing so, the effectiveness of therapy may be jeopardized. As emphasized earlier, the true test of our therapy is not how successful the children are in our clinic or therapy room, but how willing and able the children are to communicate when and where they want in their everyday environment. Reducing negative feelings, emotions, and the avoidances that result will allow for the transfer of gains into naturalistic settings and make them more resistant to relapse. A variety of techniques may be employed to help the child address feelings and emotions. These include

self-disclosure, role playing, and addressing the emotional components of the situational hierarchy.

a. Self-disclosure. This typically refers to children telling others that they stutter. It may also be accomplished through voluntary or pseudo stuttering as described earlier. With school-age children, a variety of techniques may be implemented to help them self-disclose. One approach is to comment on the stuttering after it occurs. Many children have generated the following: "Gee, I got a little stuck there. I'll have to smooth it out next time." "My stuttering is giving me a run for my money today." "Hang in there. I stutter sometimes, so the message takes a little longer to get out." "My stuttering is trying hard to boss me around." "That was one of my best stutters ever!" The content of their comment will, of course, depend upon the nature of their stuttering, their comfort level, where they are in therapy, and the context of the communicative interaction.

For school-age children who are preparing to read aloud, give a report or speech, try out for a team or club, or participate in any other public-speaking activity, we discuss the possibility of telling the audience about stuttering before they begin to speak. The speaker could inform the audience by producing some fake or pretend stuttering and then commenting on it. Some children feel comfortable after making a joke such as, "I have a 5-minute speech prepared which should take about 15 minutes if I'm lucky!" This type of comment helps to relax the speaker and the audience, and is typically interpreted as showing self-confidence and acceptance of one's stuttering.

We also discuss self-disclosure with children when they are teased or mimicked. It sometimes quiets an adversary when the child who stutters says something like, "So what if I stutter sometimes. It could be a lot worse," or "I can handle my stuttering. Too bad you can't." "If you're going to imitate me, you might as well get it right. Try this one, . . ." In our experience, children have reported that comments like these have silenced the offending child and/or brought others to the child's defense or even lightened the moment for both interactants.

Earlier in the chapter we talked about children giving presentations about stuttering in their classrooms. This is another means of letting others know that one stutters as well as educating them about how to respond. Case Example 5-4 illustrates a recent example of self-disclosure.

Case Example 5-4

Josh, a 10-year-old, established a number of contacts over electronic mail in conjunction with a school project. He had neither met any of the contacts nor spoken with them. Josh decided to let each of them know that he stutters by e-mail. He gave some examples of his own stuttering, as well as information about stuttering, and he welcomed questions. He was thrilled by the responses that included compliments concerning his willingness to share his stuttering, comments that they had learned a great deal from his message, and further questions about his experiences with and feelings about stuttering. Several respondents let Josh know that they didn't care if he stuttered, and they disclosed things about themselves that they perceived as less than ideal (e.g., overweight, uncoordinated, trouble with spelling).

---

  b. Role playing. This may be used to help a child to learn, practice, and gain confidence before trying any technique outside of the therapy environment, including those aimed at addressing emotions. Our colleague, Bill Murphy, who we mentioned previously, is famous for making movies in which he, the children, and the student clinicians play various roles in scenarios that the child who stutters has chosen. The scenarios consist of situations in which the child is having particular difficulty communicating. They do several takes, each depicting a different possible outcome to the scenario. For example, when dealing with teasing by peers, the movie might include takes during which the child says something impolite to the offender, ignores the person, or makes a comment such as those provided in the last section. Once the movie is complete, the client, Bill, and the other clinicians make popcorn and have a debut which parents, siblings, friends, or anyone else the child wishes to invite attend. This activity is a positive, creative, and enjoyable way for the child to discuss and address personal feelings. Although responses to the teasing that are not socially acceptable (e.g., saying something impolite) are not played out in reality, they are performed, discussed, and acknowledged in the movie. The child who stutters then makes a decision about which scenarios should become outtakes and which should be rehearsed further for use in real life. The result of this activity is typically the choice, additional practice, and implementation of an appropriate response to teasing.

Making phone calls is frequently a difficult context for children who stutter. Fear of the telephone and/or certain types of calls may yield avoidance of the phone and negative feelings about communication abilities and/or stuttering. By role-playing phone calls of different types and lengths, the child becomes comfortable with both the content of the calls and the techniques that will be utilized to ease stuttering and/or facilitate fluency. Developing a script and then rehearsing various types of calls with the SLP and/or others in the therapy room is used as a starting point. Gradually, "live" calls are included that are preceded by "warm-up" sessions to discuss concerns and practice techniques. Calls are made within and then outside of the therapy setting. Eventually, the child prepares for, practices, and makes calls independently outside of therapy; reports the results; and asks the SLP for assistance as needed. We have found that even our youngest school-age children want to talk on the phone to grandparents, other relatives, and their own friends, but they may be afraid to do so because of their stuttering. Thus, exploring this context in role-playing activities may be very positive and empowering for children who stutter. Some children have even used the phone to conduct surveys about stuttering, using the calls as an opportunity to gain and give information, self-disclose, and practice techniques. Case Example 5-5 contains a portion of one child's journal entry following a telephone practice session at home.

c. Emotional Components. We have already discussed the development of a situational hierarchy for examining both speaking abilities and emotions associated with stuttering. As we begin to help children to modify the feelings associated with stuttering and/or speaking, it is necessary to revisit the hierarchy continuously to determine whether feelings that were previously expressed have been maintained or changed. We engage children in a discussion that focuses on how they once felt in particular situations—whether those feelings have changed and, if so, how. By doing so, we reflect on the progress and formulate future goals.

Case Example 5-5

Barbara, a 12-year-old, had been working on making phone calls with her SLP in therapy. Before each call, she practices her easy onsets, pull-outs, and slides. Barbara had become very confident of her skills on the phone with her SLP present, but she remarked, "It's easy when you're around. I just click into my tools." Thus, she and the SLP decided that she should practice at home, just as she had in the clinic, but without her SLP. Following is Barbara's log from the experience:

October 12: After my sister and brother went to bed, I closed the door to my room and practiced my tools while reading a book for school. I made a list and decided that I would call (1) information for a phone number, (2) the public library to check on the due date for my books, (3) my friend Sabrina who talks really fast, and (4) Bruce to ask him to the Sadie Hawkins dance. I made a script for each of the calls, especially the last one! I practiced the scripts using slides at the beginning of each sentence and a pull-out on a pretend stutter, just in case. Calling information was easy and I didn't stutter. I used a slide for every sentence. When I called the library, they put me on hold and I got nervous, so I kept practicing my script. I talked pretty fast and didn't slide very much, but it came out fluent, so I felt okay. I practiced for awhile before I called Sabrina. Her mom is really sweet, so that part was easy. I couldn't use my script with Sabrina because she goes all over the place when she talks. I tried my slides a few times and did a few pull-outs, but I mostly let her talk so I wouldn't stutter too much. When I got off the phone, I was really tired, so I didn't call Bruce. I'll try again tomorrow night. Overall, it went pretty well, but I'll need a lot more practice!

C. Changing Thoughts/Attitudes

In addition to speech behaviors and feelings, a child's thoughts or attitudes about oneself, speaking, and/or stuttering will influence the way the child responds to therapeutic efforts. Thoughts and attitudes usually focus on what children perceive they can or cannot do, what they are like, and what is true or false about them in comparison with others. A child may perceive that "I can't talk," or "I'm not as good at talking as other children," or "People think I'm stupid because I stutter." These attitudes or thoughts are influenced by, and influence, the child's emotions and speech behaviors. Thus, uncovering and addressing such attitudes is an important element of fluency therapy.

1. **Identification.** As was suggested for behavioral and emotional aspects of stuttering, identifying thoughts or attitudes about oneself, others, talking, and stuttering is a starting point for addressing them.

   a. Exploring thoughts and attitudes in general. To begin, we often help children to explore their general thoughts and attitudes about themselves and about others. To do this, we use "I think" statements and encourage the child to do the same. For example, we might engage the child in a discussion about similarities and differences between boys and girls, younger and older children, friends, family members, likes/dislikes, sports, or any other topic that is appropriate to the child's age and experiences. Discussions about those things that children see themselves as doing well, and not quite as well, are also encouraged. We emphasize our interest in what the child thinks by frequently asking, "What do you think about . . . ?" We ask for more information about the experiences and/or information sources the children think are important to supporting their own point of view. We reflect their thoughts back to them to determine if we understand their viewpoints. If there are several children in a therapy group, such discussions will likely include both similarities and differences of opinion about topics. The SLP respects and encourages each child's viewpoints, acting as a model, and helps the children to question, change, and/or strengthen their perceptions. The appreciation and acceptance of individual points of view and the appropriate expression of them are also emphasized. We talk about positive and negative attitudes as well as clear and fuzzy ideas, encouraging children to think about how to change negative attitudes and clarify fuzzy thinking.

   b. Exploring thoughts and attitudes about talking and stuttering. In addition to exercises aimed at understanding and exploring general thought processes, thoughts and attitudes that pertain to talking and to stuttering are elucidated. The CAT-R is particularly helpful in this regard. Included in the CAT-R are children's perceptions of the ease or difficulty of talking (e.g., "Reading out loud in class is easy for me." "Words are hard for me to say."), the quality of or skill with which they talk (e.g., "I don't talk right." "I talk well most of the time."), and how they think others perceive their talking (e.g., "My classmates don't think I talk funny." "People don't seem to like the way I talk."). These items are helpful in stimulating discussion about children's attitudes toward talking and stuttering. Their avoidances of particular persons, situations, or speaking demands (e.g., reading, giving reports, talking on the telephone) are uncovered and discussed. As suggested earlier for identifying feelings, the strength and perceived significance of particular attitudes may also be explored. The information obtained is useful in developing, refining, and systematically addressing the child's situational hierarchy. In a group setting, we sometimes have children interview one another about their speaking abilities. This has generated some interesting and elucidating discussions among the participants. Some children who stutter have elected to conduct "man on the street" interviews to learn how others perceive their speaking abilities. This is also an opportunity to educate others about stuttering. Children who stutter often are surprised to learn that those who do not stutter have similar insecurities and concerns about their speaking abilities.

2. **Modification.** During the process of identifying thoughts and attitudes, modification of them has already begun. The SLP helps children to expand and clarify their points of view. The clinician often gently challenges the child's statements and identifies inconsistencies in what the child says and in what the child does. Case Example 5-6 illustrates how attitudes may begin to change in children who stutter.

Case Example 5-6

Eileen, an 11-year-old with whom we worked recently, thought that others perceived her, and people who stutter in general, as "stupid." After giving a report in class, she received written feedback from classmates and the teacher that indicated they perceived her to be organized, well prepared, a clear presenter, and knowledgeable. We discussed the discrepancy between her view and those of her classmates. She admitted to being surprised by the feedback, as her peers gave it anonymously. She felt that her success was a result of considerable preparation and practice of the report, and she lamented that such success was not second nature to her. We discussed the steps she would take in therapy to progress toward more natural and spontaneous use of her skills.

---

a. The first person whose attitudes need to change, if they are negative or inconsistent, is the child who stutters. The process of identifying, exploring, and discussing attitudes about self, talking, and stuttering is aimed at reinforcing positive, productive attitudes and minimizing or changing negative, destructive, or prohibitive attitudes. It is helpful to keep a written record of attitudes expressed earlier in therapy and then compare them with attitudes that emerge over time. Administering the CAT-R once or twice a year is one method of record keeping and comparison. Another is the use of a log or diary, maintained by the child, that is reviewed at appropriate junctures in therapy (e.g., at the end of each semester, school year, or more frequently if indicated by the child's progress). It is particularly important for the SLP to highlight and reinforce positive changes, helping the children to see the progress they have made and to feel good about it.

b. Oftentimes, it is also important to determine and then focus on changing the attitudes of others. This pertains to parents, teachers, siblings, peers, and additional important persons (e.g., other relatives, coaches, other professionals). Determining their attitudes may be accomplished through interviews by the SLP, completion of questionnaires or inventories, and/or observations in the home, classroom, on the playground, or in other relevant contexts. Children who are old enough, and for whom it is appropriate, may choose to interview or survey others, as mentioned earlier, to gauge attitudes about stuttering. They may do this on their own or with the participation of the SLP. Whether the SLP, child, or both obtain information about others' attitudes, the child should be actively involved in discussing what types of attitudes to expect, who might have them, how to inquire about them, the results, and how to respond to the information obtained. The child should be actively involved in planning and/or executing means for changing or augmenting attitudes that exist among those with whom the client interacts. This is an empowering experience for children who stutter and one that often results in strengthening of positive attitudes toward oneself. As was suggested for feelings about stuttering, these activities help to make stuttering a "speakable" topic, reducing the discomfort and avoidance of all involved and making it easier for the child to transfer skills into environments outside of therapy.

   c. The techniques used to help children identify and modify their own and others' attitudes are similar to those mentioned for addressing feelings. Depending upon the child, the attitudes he or she expresses and the relative weighting of behavioral, emotional, and attitudinal components, particular goals and procedures are selected. As mentioned, development, refinement, and implementation of goals formulated with the help of a situational hierarchy are key. Role-playing scenarios in which the child and others convey positive and negative attitudes about talking, stuttering, or other aspects of self may be used in a similar way to that described for emotional aspects. The child identifies key phrases that will be helpful when interacting with others, such as: "We all have things that are easier and harder for us to do. I'm working on making talking easier." "Everyone gets nervous when they have to give a speech." "We won't always agree with one another, but we should always listen."

   Presentations to classmates, teachers, parents, or others help to educate and facilitate positive attitudes. General discussions about attitudes, how they are developed, and how they change are helpful. Topics such as stereotypes, prejudices, cliques, and individual differences encourage examination of personal and societal attitudes. Materials developed by the Stuttering Foundation of America, National Stuttering Association (see Appendix C), and other organizations help the child and others understand stuttering and respond to it with positive attitudes and behaviors.

D. Group Therapy

There are many advantages to group therapy for school-age children who stutter. First, group therapy involves interaction among peers. Such interaction promotes acceptance (i.e., "I'm not alone." "It's okay to stutter.") and teamwork (i.e., "We're all in this together." "We can help one another succeed."). The group setting also allows for practice of techniques with peers and identification and discussion of differences and similarities between children and their experiences, stuttering, goals, and techniques. Children act as models for one another and enhance motivation by their support and positive interactions.

   1. Logistics. It is important that groups are composed of children of similar ages. Grouping or separating boys and girls may need to be considered. With children in kindergarten through about third grade, boys and girls typically work well together. In fourth grade, in some cases, and more so in fifth and sixth grades, boys and girls tend to grow and develop at different rates physically and exhibit enhanced awareness of gender differences. We carefully consider the individual children we are seeing before composing our groups. We also consider family composition, background, and the potential involvement of family members and/or other persons in therapy. It is also important to group children who are at similar points in therapy, even if some of their goals and achievements differ. Such differences may be used in a helpful manner whereby children assist others with skills they find easier and receive assistance and support for skills that they are still developing. Exposure to children who are significantly more advanced in development and application of skills can be motivating and rewarding; however, these types of interactions should occur at appropriate junctures in therapy, rather than continuously in a group therapy setting. An example of this might be the introduction of middle- or high-school students to fifth or sixth graders. The older students might present their own experiences with school, peers, parents, and with therapy and help to prepare the younger children as they transition to more advanced grades. We have helped to facilitate pairings between older and younger children who stutter that have blossomed outside of therapy. E-mail, telephone, and other personal contacts often develop and yield a positive and influential support system. Such relationships are also frequently the by-product of meetings between children who stutter and their families at various conferences (e.g., those sponsored by Friends of the NSA or the SFA).

2. **Establishing Goals.** Goals for individual children are first established independent of the group. As these goals are being developed, we think about other children who have similar goals and who meet the criteria specified earlier for possible grouping. Children are informed of our desire to group each of them with others, and we present our rationale for doing so. We encourage discussion of the advantages and disadvantages of group and individual therapy, focusing on the ideas, goals, and, if present, any fears or misconceptions that a child might have about each setting. Together with the child, we then specify goals that will be addressed in the group and discuss their relative importance. In some settings (e.g., school), the child (or SLP) may not have a choice about grouping. If this is the case, we fully inform the child and help in the preparation for group membership.

3. **Group Activities.** At the first group session, we ask the children to introduce themselves. With younger children (kindergarten and first graders), we ask them to give their names and those of their teachers and a little information about their families. Then we typically play an ice-breaker type of activity in which children play a game, assemble a puzzle, cooperate to construct a building with blocks, compose a mural, or so on. With older children, or with younger children who have received previous therapy, we ask them to talk about their talking, stuttering, and/or therapy experiences. If the children in the group have been in individual and/or group therapy previously, we ask them to share items from their therapy notebooks or a story about themselves (e.g., travel, favorite activities, family). This becomes a regular feature of the group and is typically called show and tell. Children present results of homework and/or bring something to show and talk about, using their therapy techniques.

Rules of the group are established during an open discussion in which all group members and the SLP participate. Once the ground rules are established, we make hard copies and add them to the children's notebooks and to the wall of the therapy room. Examples of rules include (1) Be a good listener; (2) Wait your turn; (3) Be considerate; (4) Be positive; and (5) Be a good friend. We encourage children to devise rules that are positive (i.e., "dos" rather than "don'ts"). The don'ts are discussed as the rules are formulated, but we encourage the children to think about the "right thing to do." To facilitate rule construction, we often talk about things that they have observed among children in the classroom, on the playground, and in other settings where groups are present. Both positive and negative observations are presented (and often imitated by the children). Rules are reviewed at the beginning of the first few sessions and then revisited, and revised if the children desire, every few months.

Group activities range from a focus on identifying and modifying speech behaviors; to discussing feelings and thoughts about speech, stuttering, and many other topics; to practicing skills in a variety of settings. The children devise ways of teaching skills and presenting ideas to one another with the help of the SLP. If a child has learned a technique previously, he or she becomes the leader for that presentation, soliciting assistance from other children and the SLP as needed. Such presentations are frequently practiced in individual therapy before they are conducted in the group setting when possible.

Daily activities and experiences that involve other children and/or adults are frequently discussed. Children brainstorm ways to improve communication in difficult situations and think of ways to challenge themselves to develop skills that have been mastered in easier contexts. We encourage children to give one another tips that have been helpful to them. It is important that such tips are ideas that have been tried by the child who recommends them or are ideas on which a child is currently working. Such tips are practiced in the group and then incorporated into homework assignments that the children devise. The child who generates a particular tip models the suggestion and then helps others to try it. This technique is powerful in that advice is not only given but is demonstrated. In their daily lives, children who stutter naturally receive lots of suggestions about how to talk, but fewer opportunities to learn from real-life examples. The group setting provides a unique venue for just such opportunities.

Within the group setting, children share personal goals and work to develop group goals. These are then prioritized and addressed. Children help to construct a calendar of activities, typically on a monthly basis. At the beginning of each new month, they reminisce about the previous month and plan for the next month. We incorporate current events in their homes, schools, classrooms, and elsewhere, as suggested by the children. At appropriate junctures in therapy (i.e., at the end of the semester, before a holiday break, when a child enters or leaves therapy), we have a small party at which we give awards suggested by the children (e.g., "smoothest talker," "most improved," "best ideas," "hardest worker"). In every activity, children are helped to feel that the group is theirs, particularly for older children who have had more experience with therapy. The SLP is present to contribute suggestions and materials, model and teach various skills, and provide guidelines and assistance as needed. As was suggested for individual therapy, the role of the SLP in group therapy is to provide the tools, but the children actually use them. We have found that children's perception of the group as "ours" facilitates carryover of skills and maximizes positive communicative interactions outside of the therapy setting.

IV. CONCLUSION

In this chapter, we have presented a variety of considerations and techniques for working with school-age children who stutter. As with other age groups, careful consideration is given to the relative contributions of behavioral, emotional, and attitudinal components. In contrast to therapy with preschoolers, treatment of school-age children necessitates a primary focus on the child who stutters, self-perceptions, and personal therapy goals. We see ourselves as guides, informants, supporters, coaches, and teachers, but we are not primary determiners of the child's therapy plan. Yes, we do write lesson plans, IEPs, therapy goals, procedures, and results, but these result from, rather than dictate, the child's treatment program. Likewise, others in the child's life (e.g., parents, siblings, teachers, coaches, friends, other relatives) are viewed as support personnel who are included in treatment, as befits the child's needs and goals. This does not imply that others are unimportant, but that the child holds primary responsibility and power in determining goals, activities, and progress. When this is achieved, the child is not in therapy to please or placate others but because the child wants to be there (or at least decides the need to be there). Such internal motivation will yield more significant and long-lasting effects than any external motivators (though these may be included for additional benefit). We will expand this idea further in the next chapter on therapy for adolescents and adults.

CHAPTER

6

Therapy for Adolescents and Adults

I. EXAMINING THE EVIDENCE

In Chapter 2, we outlined the essential components of a fluency assessment for both children and adults. Recall that we discussed the important diagnostic questions that need to be answered by the evaluation, and provided objectives for each. For teenagers and adults who stutter, the direction or focus of subsequent therapy should be based on (1) the nature of disfluent speech, including the frequency, proportion of different types, duration, and associated behaviors accompanying disfluencies; (2) therapy history and outcome; (3) client attitudes and beliefs about talking and stuttering; (4) client motivation for change; and (5) the level of behavioral awareness of both fluent and stuttered speech. In this chapter, we describe an integrated therapy approach that we believe addresses each of these issues and more. In Chapter 3, we discussed the primary approaches to the treatment of stuttering—fluency shaping, stuttering modification, and the integrated approach which involves both types of treatment. In the pages that follow, we discuss the specifics of this approach to the treatment of stuttering in teenagers and adults.

It has been our experience that a number of teenagers and adults who stutter have developed "learned helplessness" as a general strategy for dealing not only with their stuttering, but also in some cases with other life issues. Seligman (1998) described learned helplessness as the "giving-up reaction" (p. 15) that stems from the belief that nothing one does will matter or make a difference. In Gregory's *Controversies about Stuttering Therapy* (1979), Dean Williams writes about stuttering treatment in which he describes his "seven assumptions" about the nature of stuttering. One central assumption is that people who stutter believe their stuttering "just happens" in spite of what they do to prevent it. Williams explained that adults who stutter frequently experience an *emotional* feeling, described as anticipation or expectancy, either before or during speaking. This "feeling" motivates the individual to do something (i.e., with his speech mechanism) to keep from producing a stuttered disruption.

The things the individual does to keep from stuttering may include increasing muscular tension; holding one's breath; forcibly exhaling or inhaling; and producing head, torso, limb, and facial movements. Some of these strategies are not visible and consist of avoiding certain situations, people, speaking tasks, and the like. Over time, many people who stutter come to realize that the things they do to keep themselves from stuttering really do not help—they continue to stutter. They are aware of the feeling of anticipation and realize that, like most emotions, this feeling really does seem to "just happen" and is almost always followed by stuttering. So, over time, those who stutter come to believe that a feeling of expectancy arises and signals that stuttering will happen, and there is nothing they can do to separate the feeling they have from the stuttering they produce. Seligman (1998) might describe this type of situation as the development of an "explanatory style," a justification that we use to explain to ourselves why things happen. In the case of stuttering, many teenagers and adults who stutter develop learned helplessness because of the way in which they explain their stuttering to themselves. As a result, they may come to believe that nothing they can do will help—not even therapy. Although the person might enroll in therapy, it is with the hope that something magical will happen because that is the only way that speech will change. The result is often not just one, but a series of unsuccessful therapy experiences. The chronic pattern of experiencing a seemingly "uncontrollable" behavior (stuttering), coupled with a history of unsuccessful stuttering therapy, is the perfect recipe for learned helplessness.

According to Seligman (1998), one of the most powerful ways to address learned helplessness is to teach people that their actions have an effect, that the things they do can work. Another way to deal with learned helplessness is to teach the individual to "think differently about what caused (or causes) him to fail" (p. 67). As such, the foundation of our general philosophy of treatment for adolescents and adults who stutter is to promote self-efficacy at every level of the therapy process. We require them to be actively involved in the ongoing decision-making processes that determine the direction of their treatment. We spend a large part of therapy guiding clients in self-examination and experimentation, and we require them to set the agenda with regard to the speech strategies they want to use and the goals they want to attain. For that reason, we do not operate from a universal set of target behaviors or goals or a strict sequence of therapy tasks.

In the pages that follow, you will not see a lock-step approach to the treatment of stuttering in teenagers and adults. Instead, you will see guidelines for the important issues that may require the client's attention and your support, and the behaviors that require your skills as a teacher. It is up to the client and you to decide what to explore.

II. DEVELOPING THE TREATMENT PLAN

A. Assumptions

As mentioned, in describing his perspective on stuttering treatment, Williams (1979) discussed seven assumptions about the nature of stuttering that he believed were essential for clinicians to hold. He noted that his own orientation to stuttering therapy was based on these assumptions and that, for him, they helped to explain much of the seemingly contradictory or "unexplainable" characteristics of the behavioral development of stuttering. Most of Williams's "assumptions" are related to the attitudes and beliefs that people who stutter hold about their stuttering and their behavioral responses to these beliefs. In our own work, we have come to appreciate, as Williams did, the strong, bidirectional influence between beliefs and behaviors and that, in stuttering therapy, both must be addressed. According to Williams (1979), "In stuttering therapy, it is not a question of whether one works on both; it is a question of the ways it is done" (p. 256). The following assumptions briefly describe some of the ways in which beliefs and behaviors interact for adults and adolescents who stutter.

1. With regard to talking, the general orientation of people who stutter is "What can I do to *not stutter*?" versus "What can I do to *talk*?"

2. The behavior of stuttering is motivated by this orientation and is believed to be necessary in order to "get the word out."

3. A stuttered disruption, then, is the end result of what the person "is doing" at the present time, or "has done" to interfere with the production of normally fluent speech.

4. The motivation for the behavior described in assumption 3 is related to anticipation.

5. The "feeling" of anticipation cannot be controlled, and since stuttering usually follows, people who stutter come to believe that stuttering "just happens" (as do feelings or emotions) despite attempts to prevent "it."

6. The fears of stuttering, *although not quantifiable,* are responsible for the development of the "trying not to" or "keep from" (stuttering) response that is basic to stuttering. Four specific fears motivate the stuttering reaction pattern: (a) fear of being "found out" to be someone who stutters; (b) an inability to finish the word if one starts to stutter; (c) fear that an instance of stuttering will precipitate an "avalanche" of stuttering, making it impossible to finish the message; and (d) fear of feeling "out of control" of one's behavior.

7. While talking or preparing to talk, people who stutter attend to what they are *feeling* (i.e., emotional feelings associated with anticipation and expectancy) and not to what they are *doing* (i.e., how they are using their speech mechanism). According to Williams (1979), for people who stutter, "the 'present' is filled with emotional awareness, and is a vacuum of behavioral awareness" (p. 245).

We base much of what we do in stuttering treatment on these assumptions. Throughout the remainder of this chapter we refer to them as we describe our approach and the important issues to consider when working with teenagers and adults who stutter.

B. Getting Started: Responsibilities and Trial Therapy

As discussed in Chapter 5, treatment objectives are the who, what, when, where, why, and how of stuttering intervention. A key element in the development of a treatment plan for adults and adolescents is the clarification of responsibilities: Who is responsible for what?

1. **Client's Role.** During our initial evaluation, we have determined the nature of the client's stuttering and, to some extent, his or her beliefs and attitudes about stuttering, talking, and level of motivation. From the very first day of therapy, we try to impress upon clients that they are the experts about themselves on all aspects of speech, stuttering, attitudes, thoughts, feelings, learning style, and

so forth. Clients need to teach clinicians about themselves to help the clinician be the best coach possible. With teaching and support, the client is responsible for choosing the long-term goals for treatment and for deciding which speech strategies to practice and use. For example, we discuss with the client the options for speech goals. One person who stutters may want to use "controlled fluency" when talking; another might shoot for some "spontaneous fluency" along with "easier stuttering." Some people might decide they want to develop the ability to choose *how* they talk, depending on the situation. They want to learn ways to talk more fluently *when they want to,* and at other times "just go ahead and stutter." Whatever personal goals are set, clients must recognize that they are in control and responsible for their own learning and change.

2. **Clinician's Role.** The clinician's role can be compared with that of an athletic coach. In this regard, we are responsible for helping our clients to elicit their best to attain the goals they have established for themselves. In this way, we regard ourselves as facilitators, helping clients to explore, try different options, and select those that not only support their goals, but also make the clients feel most proficient and comfortable when using them.

3. **Trial Therapy.** Conture (1990) advocates a period of "trial" therapy for adults and adolescents who stutter, and we typically make arrangements with our clients for the first 3 to 6 weeks of therapy to constitute such a trial period. In essence, the purpose of trial therapy is to see whether the client is capable of active participation and making change, is conscientious about keeping appointments and completing assignments, and attempts to develop an attitude of "openness" about oneself and stuttering. At the end of this period of trial therapy, the clinician and the client will decide whether to continue or terminate therapy or whether to stop therapy for a short period of time and reinitiate it at a later date.

We attempt to make sure that we clearly explain what we will be looking for that will indicate to us our relationship with the client should continue. Specific observations include (1) the client's active participation in therapy sessions; (2) evidence that the client is able to make (small) behavioral changes in structured therapy tasks in the therapy room (for example, if we are working to increase accuracy of self-identification of stuttering, we want to see that the client is open and willing to attempt the task and shows some improvement over the course of several sessions); (3) the client's active participation outside of therapy, as evident from journals, logs, and completion of homework assignments; and (4) the client's overall commitment to therapy, as evidenced by keeping appointments and arriving on time.

III. MOTOR TRAINING

The integrated approach that we use includes both motor and mental training. Motor training involves the mechanics of speech and requires clients to learn, practice, and use different speech behaviors so they can talk the way they want—first by consciously attending, and then on a more automatic level. Mental training involves an active focus on thoughts, beliefs, and, to some extent, emotions. We provide training experiences in both of these areas simultaneously; as our clients are exploring ways to make speech changes, they are also reevaluating their thought processes and examining ways of actively changing the way they think in order to facilitate their newfound speech skills. Motor training is essentially composed of four major components: education, behavioral awareness, fluency skills, and stuttering modification skills.

A. Education

1. **General Information.** One goal of clinicians is to help the client develop an open attitude about stuttering. One way is by using relevant strategies from the stuttering modification (SM) approach to stuttering treatment (see Chapter 3), especially those that help the individual to reduce both the fear (see earlier discussion of Williams's "assumptions") and avoidance of both speaking and stuttering. According to Williams (1979), there are two primary strategies for dealing with fear and avoidance: confronting the behavior of stuttering and experiencing the behavior of stuttering by "stuttering openly" on at least a temporary basis. A good place to start to help the client to confront his or her own stuttering is to provide information about what stuttering is and what it is not. As described in Chapter 5, each client should have a notebook in which to keep assignments, reading materials, journal notes, and the like. We routinely provide our teenage and adult clients with "information sheets" focused on different topics of interest. For example, the following information might be contained in an information sheet that describes some of the things we know about the problem of stuttering.

   • Stuttering begins in early childhood, usually between 2 and 5 years of age.

- A large proportion of young children who stutter (anywhere from 60% to 90%) recover without therapy. When recovery occurs in these children, it typically does so within 12 to 36 months after the stuttering problem begins.
- More boys than girls develop chronic stuttering problems (about four boys for every one girl).
- The overall *prevalence* (proportion of the population exhibiting a stuttering problem at a particular point in time) is between 0.5% and 1.0%.
- The *incidence* (proportion of the population that has exhibited a stuttering problem *at any time in their life*) is approximately 4% to 5%.
- Research has shown that, *as a group,* both children and adults who stutter are more similar to, than different from, people who do not stutter. That is, they are not more likely to exhibit health, psychological, learning, communication, or mental problems. Further, as a group, the families and home environments of people who stutter are not different from those of people who do not stutter.
- A number of different speaking strategies have been shown to help people who stutter to speak more easily, almost immediately. These include speaking at a slower rate; using continuous voicing while speaking; making light or soft contact with the lips, tongue, teeth, and other places in the mouth (e.g., touching the tip of the tongue to the alveolar ridge in order to say the "t" sound); and pausing between phrases or utterances.
- Although different speaking strategies have been shown to help, many people who stutter exhibit difficulty in *consistently using* these strategies or techniques on a daily basis in different speaking situations. This is most likely related to the negative emotions, attitudes, and fears which people who stutter have learned over time as a *reaction* to their stuttering. Sometimes people who stutter also learn to use a number of behaviors to help them avoid talking and stuttering or to "escape" from stuttering. It is difficult to eliminate these kinds of coping behaviors; thus, it becomes a challenge to use the speech techniques or strategies learned in therapy. As with any behavior, motor training without mental training is not effective.

Similarly, the following are some of the things we do not know about stuttering.

- What causes stuttering to begin in the first place? It is safe to say that no one characteristic of either a child or the child's family causes stuttering. More likely, multiple risk factors are present in certain combinations, which result in the onset of stuttering in young children. Some of these risk factors include family history (heredity), gender, temperament, motor skills, overall speech and language skills, and certain aspects of the environment.

- Why do some children recover but others do not? How can we predict outcomes? We are getting better at predicting which children are likely to recover soon after the problem begins (without therapy) and which are unlikely to recover without help. This second group of children are likely to continue to stutter beyond early childhood and will need some form of therapy to learn to talk more easily. As with the cause of stuttering, usually multiple factors, present in certain combinations, will lead to early (unassisted) recovery.

- Why is there such variability in the amount of stuttering someone produces? Why can one talk easily in some situations and not in others? Why can one talk easily in a particular situation and then have a difficult time in the same situation on a different day? Speech (and stuttering) is a complex behavior. Speech behavior can easily be influenced by what one is thinking or feeling. Thus, speech (both fluent and stuttered) is similar to other relatively complex learned motor behaviors, for example, a certain golf swing, piano or guitar piece, or foul shot. We often interfere with or bungle the production of motor behaviors we have learned and can produce automatically, depending on our thoughts and feelings in a particular situation.

2. **Structure and Function of the Speech Mechanism.** Once we have discussed some of the facts about stuttering with our clients, we move to an exploration of the structure and function of the speech mechanism. Most people are relatively unfamiliar with the specific components of the speech system, including where they are and how they function, both individually and as part of a unit. After all, for most of us, speech is relatively automatic, and the key components (lungs, larynx, etc.) are not visible. Our clients are no different, and they typically show a good deal of interest in this topic. We use pictures, diagrams, models, and so forth to augment a basic description of the parts of the speech mechanism, including lungs, larynx, and speech articulators (lips, jaw, tongue, soft and hard palate, teeth, etc.).

With regard to function, we explain the ways in which we use the speech mechanism to produce normally fluent speech and how we use the same system to interfere with that process. Here is where we begin to show our clients that there is a relationship between what they do when they talk and the outcome. While explaining the *process* of speaking, we describe for our clients the parameters required for speech, and we ask them to manipulate or change those parameters individually while talking. Williams (1979) delineated these parameters as (1) airflow, (2) movement of speech articulators, (3) timing of movement, (4) degree of muscular tension, and (5) voicing. We show our clients that we use all of these parameters simultaneously when we produce smooth, fluent, forward-moving speech, and we can interrupt or interfere with that production in a number of different ways by using the same parameters. For example, if we stop airflow from the lungs, we will be unable to produce voice. If we keep our tongue pressed up behind our teeth with excessive muscle tension and for an inappropriately long period of time, then we will be able to maintain the forward flow of speech. By instructing clients to use these parameters to analyze both their fluent and stuttered speech, we are giving them the opportunity to experience, firsthand, the information we are sharing. In showing and discussing the speech mechanism with our clients, we are helping them to begin to objectify speech—to look at the process as something they do rather than as something that just happens. These discussions place the client further along the path toward "unlearning" their helplessness with regard to their stuttering.

3. **Therapy Outline and Rationale.** Another important part of the education process is to provide the client with a brief outline of therapy, along with a rationale for each of the steps. The clinician should develop a loose structure for the general direction therapy might take, and then the client and the clinician should work together to fine-tune the individual goals and tasks. The client should understand that this outline is tentative. It can, and should, change at any point during treatment, depending on the client's progress and needs. A handout may reduce the client's anxiety about expectations and will provide a reference should the client have any questions about a particular therapy activity or task. Lastly, a therapy outline prepared at the beginning of treatment will serve as a general road map for the clinician to follow.

B. Behavioral Awareness

Behavioral awareness refers to the extent to which clients can physically feel *what* they do when they stutter or interfere with speech flow, and *when* they do it. This process involves using the parameters of airflow, movement, timing, tension, and voicing to examine both fluent and stuttered or disfluent speech. It involves helping clients attend to what they are doing while speaking, rather than focusing only on what they are emotionally feeling (Williams, 1979).

Once we have explained and described the parameters we use to produce speech, we provide numerous examples of how to manipulate those parameters in our own speech. The clinician should give examples of fluent or forward-moving speech and purposeful or voluntary stuttering, and explain what he or she did with airflow, movement, and so forth, to produce them. Next, the client should be directed to perform rote speech activities, for example, counting or saying the days of the week or months of the year. These tasks almost always yield spontaneous fluency, and the clinician instructs the client to attend to what it physically feels like to produce this easy, forward-moving speech, using the terminology related to the five parameters. For example, as Robert counts from 1 to 20, the clinician directs him to attend to the way he is allowing air to flow continuously from his lungs into the oral cavity, how he is keeping the (moveable) speech articulators in continuous motion, how he is using "just the right amount" of muscular tension and timing, and so on.

When asking the client to produce purposeful stuttering, the same task can be repeated. The clinician instructs the client to examine what she is doing with airflow, voicing, and so on while producing a voluntary or purposeful stuttering. Since it is not a "real" stuttering, it is likely that the client is not experiencing the negative emotion that often accompanies genuine stuttered disruptions. The absence of this negative reaction or emotion will likely make it easier for the client to attend to what she is doing at the present time and to analyze the relationship between behavior and speech output.

The clinician and client then explore the next level of speech complexity that yields a relatively large amount of spontaneous fluency. For some people, this is oral reading. For others, it may be a simple picture description. When clients are speaking, the clinician prompts them to attend to the physical feelings associated with speaking, both fluently and disfluently. If clients produce a stuttered disruption, the clinician can ask them to stop immediately and to replicate the stuttering. We consider clients to be exhibiting a high level of behavioral awareness if they are able to produce a close imitation or purposeful stuttering. One word of caution here: It may be too confrontational for some clients if we ask them to "stutter on purpose" too soon in the treatment process. It is best to approach this slowly by making sure that the clinician has produced a good amount of purposeful stutterings first, followed by an analysis of how the speech parameters were manipulated to produce a particular utterance.

For teenagers and some adults, one good way to introduce the concept of purposeful or voluntary stuttering within the context of increasing behavioral awareness is to instruct the individual to teach the clinician how to stutter. This activity takes on the dimensions of a give-and-take interaction in that the clinician starts out by producing a purposeful stuttering and asking the client to assess his or her performance relative to the client's stuttering. The client usually ends up providing visual feedback and instruction (i.e., "No, it's more like *thththththth*is."), which the clinician immediately follows, and so on. The power of this activity is that it shows the client that the clinician is ready and willing to produce stuttered speech, and it is not only the client's behavior that is being evaluated. It also puts the client in the role of "teacher" as opposed to "student," and for some people this role reversal is empowering.

C. Fluency Skills

Working to increase behavioral awareness leads naturally into discussions about fluency skills—ways to manipulate the parameters of airflow, movement, timing, tension, and voicing to initiate and maintain fluent speech. Treatment efficacy studies have consistently shown that these techniques or strategies yield essentially fluent speech in the majority of individuals who learn to use them. While fluency skills are typically taught in a programmatic way, we use guided experimentation to allow clients to discover what fluency strategies they would like to use. As we described earlier, these strategies include the following:

- "Easy" starts or slow, physically relaxed initiation of speech and voice
- Light articulatory contact
- Prolonged speech, or increased duration of speech sounds (especially vowels) during their production
- Continuous voicing (attention paid to keeping the voice "on" while speaking)

- Phrasing and pausing, making sure to use continuous voicing to connect the sounds and words within each phrase

The clinician needs to provide ample demonstration of each strategy and allow the client to practice each one alone and in combination. This practice should be done using the same general principles that speech-language pathologists use to teach any new behavior; that is, practice the new behavior in speech stimuli of increasing complexity (syllables, words, phrases, sentences, and so on) both in and out of the therapy room. At first, the clinician should model the strategies in an exaggerated manner, resulting in fluent speech that is extremely slow and laborious sounding. This allows the client to grasp the basic behaviors and practice them in an unhurried fashion. It is essential that once clients are successful in using the fluency skills, the clinician helps them to increase the speed of production (essentially, their speaking rate), and in other ways shape the fluency to approximate more normal-sounding speech.

It is important to involve clients in the decision-making process. At some point, they will need to decide which strategy or bundle of strategies to focus on in therapy. The clinician guides the selection process by helping the client to self-evaluate. What strategies help to produce the most fluent speech? What strategies "feel" right; which ones do I feel comfortable using? It is likely the strategies that feel most comfortable are those the client believes yield relatively natural-sounding speech and do not compromise spontaneity of communication to use. In our experience, the client's active participation in the selection of strategies to use increases the probability of both transfer and maintenance. This can be especially true for teenagers, who sometimes prefer the old familiar behavior of stuttering with which their listeners are familiar, to the "new" way of talking, which might be fluent, but which listeners' perceive as a different way of speaking for the client.

D. Stuttering Modification

1. **Identification.** As previously discussed, we advocate an integrated approach to the treatment of stuttering, one that emphasizes both fluency skills and the identification and modification of stuttering. Many clients learn to use fluency skills to the point that their conversational speech is relatively stutter free, both in and outside of the clinic. Being able to do so goes a long way to reduce the fear of stuttering; however, it is our practice to also provide the client with tools for modifying the behavior of stuttering as an additional strategy for reducing the fear of both stut-

tering and speaking. Being armed with the ability to initiate and maintain fluency and to problem-solve ways to change a stuttered disruption quickly offers the client a complete toolbox for coping with stuttering.

To accomplish this, we teach fluency and stuttering modification skills simultaneously. We attempt to help the client to recognize that one approach is not essentially better than the other, but that they complement each other.

Clients' work to increase their behavioral awareness of the process of speaking paves the way for the first step in learning how to modify stuttering: identification. Because of the activities used to teach behavioral awareness, clients are experienced in attending to what they are doing when speaking. The focus on identification refines this process. In addition, identification is a powerful tool to desensitize clients toward stuttering. Our identification work is based on the techniques developed by Conture (1990), and it includes both off-line and on-line identification of stuttered disruptions. The terminal goal for this sort of work is that clients will be able to feel themselves starting to interfere with the forward flow of speech physically, and they will modify or change their behavior either before or during the stuttered disruption. This modification may result in either fluent speech or shorter, less effortful, and physically less tense instances of stuttering. Ultimately, the identification and modification sequence will become fairly automatic. A helpful analogy to use is one of riding a bicycle and starting to fall over. It is usually the case that one immediately senses (physically and cognitively) and identifies that he or she is falling over and, just as quickly, initiates a series of physical behaviors to become upright again. This all takes place in a matter of milliseconds, and the person does not have to think about the process. Instead, the rider senses a disruption and modifies behavior accordingly by attending to the kinesthetic and proprioceptive correlates of falling, and then self-correcting. In many ways, we hope that the process of stuttering modification will mirror this process.

a. Off-line identification. Identification usually begins off-line, where the client identifies stuttering in audio- or videotaped speech samples. A good place to start is with others' speech samples, including the clinician's purposeful stuttering, and move to identification of stuttering from taped samples of the client's speech. The abilities and sensitivity of the client will determine where the clinician begins. For some clients, having to listen to and identify stuttering in their own speech feels too threatening early on in the therapy process. For these individuals, it is best to spend time listening to and identifying stuttering in the speech of other speakers.

In off-line identification tasks, clients are instructed to raise a finger as soon as they hear or see the speaker on the audio- or videotape begin to interfere. The clinician must make the most of teaching opportunities here; that is, when the client identifies a stuttered disruption, the clinician can attempt to replicate the disfluency and ask the client for feedback. The client should then be instructed to replicate the disfluency and should also be prompted to use fluency skills to produce the word more easily. In addition, the clinician can ask the client to show how one might produce the disfluency under analysis and then change it into a form of easier stuttering.

b. On-line identification. When clients become proficient in off-line identification of their disfluencies, then it is time to move to on-line identification. This involves identifying real-life stuttering, either in clients' speech or in the speech of someone with whom they are speaking. The objective is to identify quickly, so that if clients are identifying stuttering in their speech, it is done early on in the process, giving the clients enough time to make changes. Typically, the clinician will start by asking clients to identify stuttering in the clinician's speech while reading, describing a picture, or engaging in a brief, structured conversation with the client. The instructions to clients are to "raise your finger as soon as you see or hear me beginning to interfere (or to stutter)." This particular task provides the client with many opportunities to see the clinician "stutter on purpose," and, in doing so, it assists in the continued development of a trusting and open clinician-client relationship.

Once clients can quickly and accurately identify stuttering in the speech of others on-line, they move to the identification of their own stuttering while speaking. This task can be extremely difficult for the client, not just because of the level of attending required, but also because the focus of attention and analysis is on the client's stuttering, something the client has probably worked long and hard to suppress. If the clinician has accurately gauged the client's level of sensitivity, and has brought this person slowly to this point in therapy with lots of support, then the move to on-line identification should go smoothly. An important point here is that with on-line identification, the client instructions change. Rather than directing clients to identify stuttering as soon as they hear or see it, the instruction should be to "raise your finger as soon as you feel yourself beginning to interfere." As clients become proficient at doing this, there are again many opportunities for practicing stuttering modification. For example, the clinician can tell clients beforehand that he or she will instruct them to replicate their behavior after the accurate identification of a specified number of stuttered disruptions. This process can be followed immediately by experimentation on how the client might change that (now purposeful) stuttering behavior, and the process can be repeated and practiced.

2. **Purposeful or Voluntary Stuttering.** As discussed, stuttering on purpose can be a good tool for desensitization, and it can also serve as an important bridge between the identification and modification of actual stutterings. Used in conjunction with on-line identification, voluntary stuttering gives clients the opportunity to focus on their speech, to physically attend to when and how they stutter, and to experience the outcome of that physical feeling immediately through replication of the identified stuttering. Following this, clients can experiment with ways to manipulate purposeful stuttering. Repeated practice of this sequence—identification to replication (purposeful stuttering) to modification—is essential.

3. **Modification.** The modification, or change, of stuttered disruptions involves consideration of the same five parameters of speech as discussed earlier. When one interferes with the forward flow of speech—in the form of stuttering—what parameter or combination of parameters needs to be changed to continue to move forward in a smooth manner? Airflow? Tension? Timing? Here is where clients, with their clinician's guidance and feedback, need to attend to how their stuttered disruptions differ from their fluent speech in terms of these speech parameters. Some possible examples include:

- Initiate airflow and voicing and "slide out" of the disfluency into the next sound.

- Slowly decrease the physical tension, initiate airflow and voicing, and "slide out."
- Practice "holding on" to a moment of stuttering. At some point, the client will have to change the actual stuttering to a purposeful disfluency in order to continue to produce it. Soon after, the client should practice modifying the purposeful stuttering in the above ways.

4. **Practice, Practice, Practice.** A key factor in learning any motor skill is practice. This cannot be emphasized enough. For the new way of speaking to become the dominant pattern, it has to be practiced often, and the client needs to receive appropriate levels and types of feedback and reinforcement from the clinician. In addition, the client needs to engage in self-practice and evaluation on a daily basis.

IV. MENTAL TRAINING

Motor training alone might help one to acquire a new behavior or behaviors, but it is not enough if one wants to be able to use that behavior consistently in everyday situations. We include a mental training component in our approach to stuttering treatment. In addition to addressing the stuttering-related counseling issues that clients typically present, it is important to assist them in becoming consciously aware of how specific patterns of thought affect both their stuttering and their performance in using fluency and stuttering modification strategies. To do so, we have adopted some of the strategies used by sports psychologists (Waite, 1997) and specialists in motivational work and leadership training. In general, mental training consists of three main components: cognitive restructuring; visualization or guided imagery; and relaxation, or specifically, the relaxation response (Benson, 1975).

A. Cognitive Restructuring

Cognitive restructuring refers to a general exploration of thoughts, feelings, and beliefs, followed by a reality assessment. It is helpful for the clinician to instruct clients to focus on what they think, feel, and believe about their stuttering as it relates to particular situations, people, and events and then to contrast those projections with what really happened or happens. For some clients, a journal is a good place to record this comparison. They should note particular thoughts and feelings surrounding an upcoming or frequently occurring speaking situation and then immediately record the outcome of the situation (in most cases this will be some sort of assessment of stuttering). How did the reality of the situation compare with what the client thought or believed would happen? In many cases, the client's expectations about the situation are not matched by the reality. Sometimes these expectations are better, but sometimes they are worse than what really happens. At any rate, frequent reality checks help clients to attend to their thoughts and emotions and the extent to which they reflect the actual experience.

Paying attention to how one thinks and feels also helps to bring negative or self-defeating self-talk to one's consciousness. What things do clients tell themselves as they approach certain speaking situations or after stuttering? Along with assessing the relationship between thoughts, beliefs, and outcome, the clinician can assist clients in developing, practicing, and choosing to use positive self-talk. With the clinician's guidance, clients should develop positive self-messages that are particularly meaningful to them and practice using these at times when negative thoughts take hold. Waite (1997) recommends a strategy called "stoppage" to modify self-defeating self-talk. She advocates merely saying "STOP," either aloud when possible or loudly to oneself. This should be followed by a deep breath and then a "letting go" of criticism and doubt. This "stoppage" and deep, cleansing breath should become a cue for choosing to use positive self-talk (e.g., "I have important things to say," "I know I'm okay," or whatever appears to be most helpful to the individual). According to Waite, it is important to use thought "stoppage" as many times as it takes. Eventually clients will use it less and less as they silence the internal critic and break the cycle of negative thought and emotion.

Additional methods for cognitive restructuring include:

- Be in the present moment, not in the past or future.
- Accept without evaluation, then refocus.
- Choose to trust yourself, your abilities, and your training; trust allows motor abilities to surface.

B. Visualization or Guided Imagery

Visualization is the process of forming images or pictures in one's mind of best performances. These images can be visual (what the experience would look like to someone watching us), kinesthetic (how one's body feels during the experience), auditory (how the experience sounds), tactile (how things feel to the touch), and even emotional (what emotional state is one in during the experience). Adolescents and adults who stutter can repeatedly call up images of themselves talking easily in various contexts, and doing so builds experience and confidence in their ability to handle any situation. When they mentally practice this particular skill, their minds and bodies become better prepared to perform the skill. The goal is to create a vivid and real speaking image with complete control over what happens.

C. Relaxation

Many adults and teenagers who stutter derive benefit from receiving training in relaxation methods. When we approach this issue with our clients, we make sure to convey the message that the problem of stuttering is not caused by pervasive tension or anxiety, but that these factors may contribute to increased amounts of stuttering. In addition, we advocate relaxation training, because regular use of such methods may help the client to maintain a clearer focus in therapy.

The two primary types of relaxation are physical and mental. To attain a state of physical or muscular relaxation, we use a variation of Jacobson's *Progressive Relaxation* (1938), in which the person alternately tenses and relaxes specific muscle groups, starting at the feet and progressively moving up the body. This technique helps the client to experience not only the differences between static states of muscular tension and relaxation, but also the transition between these two states. We want the client to develop behavioral awareness of this feeling of changing from a state of muscular tension to one of relaxation or "looseness," because it is similar to what it feels like to change a moment of tense and struggled stuttering into an easier, more relaxed form of speech (dis)fluency. We emphasize to our clients that learning a technique for producing physical relaxation helps them to develop an overall increase in "body awareness" that ultimately helps them to make speech changes.

To attain a state of mental relaxation, we teach Benson's (1975) version from *The Relaxation Response*. Benson, a cardiologist, developed the relaxation response to help his patients deal with stress through reducing their heart rate and blood pressure. To do this, a person needs to spend time each day in a comfortable position in a quiet environment. During this time, the individual adopts a passive, "let it happen" attitude, and with eyes closed, he or she uses a mental device to help focus the mind during quiet breathing. This mental device is a short word or phrase which is repeated silently during slow exhalations. This passive attitude is essential in helping the person to disregard passing thoughts and refocus on the here and now (in the form of breathing). The relaxation response, then, is the physiological consequence of this practice. It includes a reduced heart rate and breathing rate and an overall lower metabolism. The related mental benefits from these body changes include increased clarity of thought and decreased "time urgency" or reduction of the feeling that we need to rush. It is this reduction in the feeling of being rushed to action, especially to communicate verbally, that is helpful to people who stutter. The feeling that it is okay to take your time to speak can facilitate speech fluency as well as easy stuttering.

V. CONCLUSION

In this chapter, we have provided the key components of an integrated approach to the treatment of stuttering in teenagers and adults. We focused our discussion on ways to facilitate changes in the behavioral and attitudinal factors underlying stuttering, because these tend to be more generic in nature. The clients' emotional responses to their stuttering are more likely to be unique, and they need to be uncovered and addressed using standard counseling techniques.

APPENDIX

A

Daily Stuttering Tracking Form Rater: _____

DATE	RATE TODAY FROM 0–8 0 = NO STUTTERING 8 = VERY SEVERE STUTTERING	COMMENTS AND QUESTIONS
	0 1 2 3 4 5 6 7 8	
	0 1 2 3 4 5 6 7 8	
	0 1 2 3 4 5 6 7 8	
	0 1 2 3 4 5 6 7 8	
	0 1 2 3 4 5 6 7 8	
	0 1 2 3 4 5 6 7 8	
	0 1 2 3 4 5 6 7 8	
	0 1 2 3 4 5 6 7 8	
	0 1 2 3 4 5 6 7 8	
	0 1 2 3 4 5 6 7 8	
	0 1 2 3 4 5 6 7 8	
	0 1 2 3 4 5 6 7 8	

A P P E N D I X

B

Speaking Situation Analysis Form

SITUATION	COMMENTS	RANK

APPENDIX

C

Stuttering Resources

ASHA Special Interest Division 4: Fluency and Fluency Disorders: "Vision—excellence of research in fluency and fluency disorders and of service to those who stutter; recognition of the multidimensionality of Fluency Disorders; public awareness and understanding of Fluency Disorders and acceptance of those with chronic stuttering and universal access to a cadre of specialists in the prevention and treatment of Fluency Disorders." (quotation from ASHA website)

Contact Information

Telephone
ASHA Action Center
800-498-2071

Coordinator
    Nan E. Bernstein Ratner, Ph.D., CCC-SLP
    University of Maryland
    Dept. of Hearing and Speech Sciences
    0100 Lefrak Hall
    College Park, MD 20817

Website
    http://professional.asha.org/sidivisions/sid_4.htm

National Stuttering Association: "Since 1977, The National Stuttering Association has provided hope, help, education, and empowerment for these people through its local support groups, publications, annual convention, and workshops for people who stutter, parents, teachers, and speech-language professionals." (quotation from website)

Contact Information

Telephone
    800-364-1677

Fax
    714-693-7554

Postal address
    5100 East La Palma, Suite 208
    Anaheim Hills, CA 92807

Website
    http://www.nsastutter.org/

Electronic mail
    nsastutter@aol.com

Friends: The Association of Young People Who Stutter: "FRIENDS is a national organization created to provide a network of love and support for children and teenagers who stutter, their families, and the professionals who work with them." (quotation from website)

Contact Information
Website
http://www.friendswhostutter.org/

Electronic mail
LCaggiano@aol.com

Stuttering Foundation of America: "The Stuttering Foundation of America, the first nonprofit, charitable association in the world to concern itself with the prevention and improved treatment of stuttering, distributes over a million publications to the public and professionals each year. They provide information for those who stutter and their families as well as professionals." (quotation from website)

Contact Information

Telephone
800-992-9392
901-452-7343

Fax
901-452-3931

Postal address
3100 Walnut Grove Road, Suite 603
P.O. Box 1174
Memphis, TN 38111-0749

Website
http://www.stuttersfa.org/

Electronic mail
stutter@vantek.net

The Stuttering Homepage: This site was created by Judith Kuster, a professor at Mankato State University, Minnesota. It contains extensive information, references, links, chat rooms, conference information, and other resources for people who stutter; professionals who treat them; and students, parents, and others seeking knowledge about or assistance with stuttering.

Contact Information

Website
http://www.mankato.msus.edu/dept/comdis/kuster/stutter.html

REFERENCES

Adams, M. R. (1974). A physiologic and aerodynamic interpretation of fluent and stuttered speech. *Journal of Fluency Disorders, 1,* 35–47.

Ambrose, N. G., & Yairi, E. (1999). Normative disfluency data for early childhood stuttering. *Journal of Speech, Language, & Hearing Research, 42*(4), 895–909.

Andrews, G., & Cutler, J. (1974). Stuttering therapy: The relation between changes in symptom level and attitudes. *Journal of Speech & Hearing Disorders, 39,* 312–319.

Benson, H. (1975). *The relaxation response.* New York: W. Morrow & Co., Inc.

Bloodstein, O. (1975). Stuttering as tension and fragmentation. In J. Eisenson (Ed.), *Stuttering: A second symposium.* New York: Harper & Row.

Bloodstein, O. (1995). Theories of stuttering. In O. Bloodstein (Ed.), *A handbook on stuttering* (5th ed., pp. 59–104). San Diego: Singular Publishing Group.

Brutten, G. & Dunham, S. (1989). The Communication Attitude Test: A normative study of grade school children. *Journal of Fluency Disorders, 14,* 371–377.

Conture, E. G. (Ed.). (1990). *Stuttering* (2nd ed.). Englewood Cliffs, NJ: Prentice Hall.

Conture, E. G. (1997). Evaluating childhood stuttering. In R. Curlee & G. Siegel (Eds.), *Nature and treatment of stuttering: New directions* (2nd ed., pp. 239–256). Boston: Allyn & Bacon.

Conture, E. G. (2001). *Stuttering: Its nature, diagnosis, and treatment.* Boston: Allyn & Bacon.

Cooper, E. B., & Cooper, C. S. (1985). *Personalized fluency control therapy.* Allen, TX: DLM.

Cooper, E. B., & Cooper, C. S. (1995). *Cooper assessment for stuttering syndromes: Children's version.* San Antonio: The Psychological Corporation.

Culatta, R., & Goldberg, S. A. (1995). Synopsis of approaches to the treatment of stuttering. In R. Culatta & S. A. Goldberg (Eds.), *Stuttering therapy: An integrated approach to theory and practice* (pp. 209–257). Needham Heights, MA: Allyn & Bacon.

Denham, S. A., Mitchell-Copeland, J., Strandberg, K., Auerbach, S., & Blair, K. (1997). Parental contributions to preschoolers' emotional competence: Direct and indirect effects. *Motivation and Emotion, 21*(1), 65–86.

DeNil, L. F., and Brutten, G. J. (1991). Speech-associated attitudes of stuttering and non-stuttering children. *Journal of Speech and Hearing Research, 34,* 60–66.

Granowsky, A., Cartier, N., & Bettoli, D. (1996). *The tortoise and the hare, friends at the end (Another point of view).* Raintree/Steck-Vaughn.

Guitar, B. (1997). Therapy for children's stuttering and emotions. In R. Curlee & G. Siegel (Eds.), *Nature and treatment of stuttering: New directions* (2nd ed., pp. 280–291). Boston: Allyn & Bacon.

Guitar, B. (1998). *Stuttering: An integrated approach to its nature and treatment* (2nd ed.). Baltimore: Williams & Wilkins.

Guitar, B. (1999). *The child who stutters: Practical advice for the school setting* (video). Available from the Stuttering Foundation of America, 3100 Walnut Grove Road, Suite 603, Memphis, TN 38111-0749.

Guitar, B. & Bass, C. (1978). Stuttering therapy: The relation between attitude change and long-term outcome. *Journal of Speech and Hearing Disorders, 43,* 392–400.

Guitar, B., Kopff-Schaefer, H., Donahue-Kilburg, G., & Bond, L. (1992). Parent verbal interaction and speech rate. *Journal of Speech & Hearing Research, 35*(4), 742–754.

Ham, R. (1990). *Therapy of stuttering: Preschool through adolescence.* Englewood Cliffs, NJ: Prentice Hall.

Ingham, J., & Riley, J. (1998). Guidelines for documentation of treatment efficacy for young children who stutter. *Journal of Speech, Language, & Hearing Research, 40,* 753–770.

Jacobson, E. (1938). *Progressive relaxation; a physiological and clinical investigation of muscular states and their significance in psychology and medical practice* (2nd ed.). Chicago: The University of Chicago Press.

Johnson, W. (1967). Stuttering. In W. Johnson, and D. Moeller, (Eds.) *Speech Handicapped School Children* (3rd edition). New York: Harper & Row. pp. 229–329.

Johnson, W., & associates. (1959). *The onset of stuttering.* Minneapolis: University of Minnesota Press.

Johnson, W., Darley, F. L., & Spriestersbach, D. C. (1963). *Diagnostic methods in speech pathology.* New York: Harper & Row.

Kelly, E. M. (under review). The effects of parental speech rate modification on the speech rates and fluency of children who stutter. Submitted to *Journal of Speech, Language, and Hearing Research.*

Kelly, E. M. (1994). Speech rates and turn-taking behaviors of children who stutter and their fathers. *Journal of Speech & Hearing Research, 37*(6), 1284–1294.

Kelly, E., & Conture, E. (1992). Speaking rates, response time latencies, and interrupting behaviors of young stutterers, nonstutterers, and their mothers. *Journal of Speech & Hearing Research, 35*(6), 1256–1267.

Kent, R. D. (1984). Stuttering as a temporal programming disorder. In R. F. Curlee & W. H. Perkins (Eds.), *Nature and treatment of stuttering: New directions* (pp. 283–302). San Diego: College-Hill Press.

LaSalle, L. R., & Conture, E. G. (1995). Disfluency clusters of children who stutter: Relation of stutterings to self-repairs. *Journal of Speech & Hearing Research, 38,* 965–977.

Luterman, D. M. (1996). *Conseling persons with communication disorders and their families* (3rd ed.). Austin, TX: Pro-Ed.

Masterson, J. J., & Kamhi, A. G. (1991). The effects of sampling conditions on sentence production in normal, reading-disabled, and language-learning-disabled children. *Journal of Speech & Hearing Research, 34*(3), 549–558.

Murphy, W. P. (1999a). *The school clinician: Ways to be more effective* (video). Available from the Stuttering Foundation of America, 3100 Walnut Grove Road, Suite 603, Memphis, TN 38111-0749.

Murphy, W. P. (1999b). *The school-age child who stutters: Dealing effectively with guilt and shame.* Memphis: Stuttering Foundation of America.

Paden, E., & Yairi, E. (1996). Phonological characteristics of children whose stuttering persisted or recovered. *Journal of Speech & Hearing Research, 39,* 987–990.

Paden, E., Yairi, E., & Ambrose, N. (1999). Early childhood stuttering II: Initial status of phonological abilities. *Journal of Speech, Language, & Hearing Research, 42*(5), 1113–1124.

Perkins, W., Rudas, J., Johnson, L., & Bell, J. (1976). Stuttering: Dis-coordination of phonation with articulation and respiration. *Journal of Speech and Hearing Research, 19,* 509–522.

Ramig, P. (1999.) *The school clinician: Ways to be more effective* (video). Available from the Stuttering Foundation of America, 3100 Walnut Grove Road, Suite 603, Memphis, TN 38111-0749.

Riley, G. (1981). *Stuttering prediction instrument for young children* (3rd ed.). Austin, TX: Pro-Ed.

Riley, G. (1994). *Stuttering severity instrument for young children (SSI-3)* (3rd ed.). Austin, TX: Pro-Ed.

Schum, R. L. (1986). *Counseling in speech and hearing practice.* Rockville, MD: National Student Speech Language Hearing Association, Clin. Series No. 9.

Schwartz, H. D. (1999). *A primer for stuttering therapy.* Needham Heights, MA: Allyn & Bacon.

Seligman, M. E. P. (1998). *Learned optimism: How to change your mind and your life.* New York: Simon & Schuster, Inc.

Shapiro, D. A. (1999). *Stuttering intervention: A collaborative journey to fluency freedom.* Austin, TX: Pro-Ed.

Sheehan, J. (1958). Conflict theory of stuttering. In J. Eisenson (Ed.), *Stuttering: A symposium* (pp. 121–166). New York: Harper & Row.

Siegel, G. M. (1998). Stuttering: Theory, research, and therapy. In A. K. Cordes & R. J. Ingham (Eds.), *Treatment efficacy for stuttering: A search for empirical bases* (pp. 103–114). San Diego: Singular Publishing Group.

Siegel, G. M. (1999). Integrating affective, behavioral, and cognitive factors. In N. B. Ratner & E. C. Healey (Eds.), *Stuttering research and practice: Bridging the gap* (pp. 115–122). Mahwah, NJ: Lawrence Erlbaum Associates.

Smith, A. (1999). Stuttering: A unified approach to a multifactorial, dynamic disorder. In N. Bernstein-Ratner & E. C. Healey (Eds.), *Stuttering research and practice: Bridging the gap* (pp. 27–44). Mahwah, NJ: Lawrence Erlbaum Associates.

Smith, A., & Kelly, E. (1997). Stuttering: A dynamic multifactorial model. In R. F. Curlee & G. M. Siegel (Eds.), *Nature and treatment of stuttering: New directions* (2nd ed., pp. 204–217). Needham Heights, MA: Allyn & Bacon.

Starkweather, C. W. (1997). Learning and its role in stuttering development. In R. F. Curlee & G. M. Siegel (Eds.), *Nature and treatment of stuttering: New directions* (2nd ed., pp. 79–95). Needham Heights, MA: Allyn & Bacon.

Starkweather, C. W., Gottwald, S. R., & Halfond, M. H. (1990). *Stuttering prevention: A clinical method.* Englewood Cliffs, NJ: Prentice Hall.

Stephenson-Opsal, D., & Bernstein-Ratner, N. (1988). Maternal speech rate modification and childhood stuttering. *Journal of Fluency Disorders, 13*(1), 49–56.

Throneburg, R. N., & Yairi, E. (2001). Durational, proportionate, and absolute frequency characteristics of disfluencies: A longitudinal study regarding persistence and recovery. *Journal of Speech, Language, & Hearing Research, 44*(1), 38–51.

Van Riper, C. (1973). *The treatment of stuttering.* Englewood Cliffs, NJ: Prentice Hall.

Van Riper, C. (1982). *The nature of stuttering* (2nd ed.). Englewood Cliffs, NJ: Prentice Hall.

Waite, B. T. (1997). Personal communication. *www.psyww.com/mtsite.*

Wall, M. J., & Myers, F. L. (1995). A review of therapies. In M. J. Wall & F. L. Myers (Eds.), *Clinical management of childhood stuttering* (2nd ed., pp. 195–238). Austin, TX: Pro-Ed.

Watkins, R. V., Yairi, E., & Ambrose, N. G. (1999). Early childhood stuttering III: Initial status of expressive language abilities. *Journal of Speech, Language, & Hearing Research, 42*(5), 1125–1135.

Williams, D. E. (1979). A perspective on approaches to stuttering therapy. In H. Gregory (Ed.), *Controversies about stuttering therapy* (pp. 241–268). Baltimore: University Park Press.

Williams, D. E. (1982). Coping with attitudes and beliefs about stuttering. *Journal of Childhood Communication Disorders, 6*(1), 60–66.

Williams, D. E., & Silverman, F. H. (1968). Note concerning articulation of school-age stutterers. *Perceptual Motor Skills, 27,* 713–714.

Williams, D. E., Silverman, F. H., & Kools, J. A. (1968). Disfluency behavior of elementary-school stutterers and nonstutterers: The adaptation effect. *Journal of Speech & Hearing Research, 11,* 622–630.

Wingate, M. E. (1962). Evaluation and stuttering. Part 1: Speech characteristics of young children. *Journal of Speech & Hearing Disorders, 27,* 106–115.

Wingate, M. E. (1964). A standard definition of stuttering. *Journal of Speech Hearing Disorders, 29,* 484–489.

Wingate, M. E. (1984). Stuttering as a prosodic disorder. In R. F. Curlee & W. H. Perkins (Eds.), *Nature and treatment of stuttering: New directions* (2nd ed., pp. 215–235). San Diego: College-Hill Press.

Yairi, E. (1997). Home environments and parent-child interaction in childhood stuttering. In R. Curlee & G. Siegel (Eds.), *Nature and treatment of stuttering: New directions* (2nd ed., pp. 22–48). Boston: Allyn & Bacon.

Yairi, E. (1999). Epidemiologic factors and stuttering research. In N. Bernstein-Ratner & E. C. Healey (Eds.), *Stuttering research and practice: Bridging the gap* (pp. 45–53). Mahwah, NJ: Lawrence Erlbaum Associates.

Yairi, E., & Ambrose, N. G. (1999). Early childhood stuttering I: Persistency and recovery rates. *Journal of Speech, Language, & Hearing Research, 42*(5), 1097–1112.

Zebrowski, P. M. (1999). *Counseling parents of children who stutter.* Memphis: Stuttering Foundation of America.

Zebrowski, P. M. (2000). Stuttering. In J. B. Tomblin, H. L. Morris, & D. C. Spriestersbach (Eds.), *Diagnosis in Speech-Language Pathology* (2nd ed., pp. 199–231). San Diego: Singular Publishing Group.

Zebrowski, P. M., & Cilek, T. D. (1997). Stuttering therapy in the elementary school setting: Guidelines for clinician-teacher collaboration. *Seminars in Speech & Language, 18*(4), 329–340.

Zebrowski, P. M., & Schum, R. L. (1993). Counseling parents of children who stutter. *American Journal of Speech-Language Pathology, 2*(2), 65–73.

Zebrowski, P. M., Weiss, A., Savelkoul, E., & Hammer, C. S. (1996). The effect of maternal rate reduction on the stuttering, speech rates, and linguistic productions of children who stutter: Evidence from individual dyads. *Clinical Linguistics & Phonetics, 10*(3), 189–206.

Zimmermann, G. (1980). Stuttering: A disorder of movement. *Journal of Speech & Hearing Research, 23,* 122–136.

INDEX

Speech
  physically relaxed initiation of, 129
  prolonged, 129
Speech articulators, 126
Speech behavior, 126
  changing, 94–101
Speech disfluency
  in adults, 27–32
  average duration of, 14–15
  average frequency of, 13
  in children, 20–21. *See also*
  clustered, 14
  describing and measuring, 12–13, 27–29
  type of, 13–14
  what is?, 5–6
  See also Stutter-like disfluencies (SLDs)
Speech fluency, 4–5
Speech-language pathologist (SLP), 40–41
Speech mechanism, structure and function
    of, 126–127
Speech rate, 17, 23, 67–69
Spontaneous fluency, 94, 123
Spriestersbach, D. C., 16, 148
Starkweather, C. W., 19, 149
Stephenson-Opsal, D., 68, 149
Sticky vs. smooth, 72–73
Strandberg, K., 102, 147
Stretched speech, 99. *See also* Prolonged
    speech
Stretchy speech, 73
Stuttered disruption, 122, 133–134
Stuttering
  assessment of. *See* Assessment of
    stuttering
  as behavior, 3–4
  causes of, 125–126
  definitions of, 1–7
  as disorder, 1–3
  identifying, 95–97. *See also*
    Identification
  severity of, 16
*Stuttering: An Integrated Approach to Its
    Nature and Treatment*, 37
Stuttering Foundation of America (SFA),
    52, 113, 145

Stuttering Homepage, 146
Stuttering modification (SM) therapy, 39,
    86, 124
  identification for, 130–133
  techniques, 99–100
*Stuttering Prediction Instrument for Young
    Children* (SPI), 16
Stuttering resources, 143–146
*Stuttering Severity Instrument for Children
    and Adults—3* (SSI-3), 16
*Stuttering Therapy: An Integrated
    Approach to Theory and
    Practice*, 37
Stuttering tracking form, 60, 139–140
Stutter-like disfluencies (SLDs), 6–7. *See
    also* Speech disfluency
"Stutter more fluently" approach, 39–40

T

Talking, adults' beliefs about, 30–32
Teachers
  in elastic band exercise, 73–74
  role of, 60, 90–94
Teasing, 93
Telephone calls, 108
Tension, element of, 68
Therapy
  as indicated, 50–54
  decisions, based on evaluation results,
    50–54
Therapy outline, 127
Thoughts
  changing children's, 109–113
  speech behavior and, 126
Throneburg, R. N., 51, 56, 149
Time, element of, 67–68
Topic contextualization, 25
Tortoise and the Hare, The, 72
Tracking form, 139–140
Treatment objectives, 87–94
Treatment plan
  for adults, 121–124
  for children, 22–27, 85–94
  developing, 54–66
Trial therapy, 123–124